Reset Your Clock

Mastering Sleep Solutions for Circadian Rhythm Disorders

Well-Being Publishing

Contents

Introduction

Sleep is not just a nightly event. It is a timed biological process shaped by light, routine, movement, meals, and the pressure to stay alert or rest at specific hours. When those signals line up, sleep tends to arrive more easily and daytime energy feels steadier. When they do not, the result can be a body that feels tired at the wrong time, wired at night, and out of sync with the demands of daily life.

That mismatch is the central problem in circadian rhythm sleep disorders. The issue is not simply that someone is sleeping too little or too much. It is that the timing of sleep is drifting away from the timing that the brain and body are trying to follow. A person may have enough opportunity to sleep yet still feel unable to fall asleep until very late, wake too early, or struggle to remain alert when they need to function. The clock is running, but not in a way that matches the schedule.

This matters because the circadian system influences far more than sleep onset. It helps regulate alertness, digestion, body temperature, hormone release, reaction time, and mood. That means a misaligned clock can show up as more than insomnia. It can appear as morning grogginess, evening energy surges, difficulty concentrating, changes in appetite, irritability, and a sense that the body is always a few hours behind or ahead of the day.

Many people spend years trying to force sleep by going to bed earlier, sleeping in later, or pushing through with caffeine and willpower. Those strategies may temporarily help with exhaustion, but they rarely correct the underlying timing problem. In fact, they can sometimes make the pattern harder to recognize by masking the real rhythm of the body. A more effective approach begins with understanding what the clock is doing and how it can be shifted in a controlled way.

Resetting the clock is not about making the body obey a rigid schedule through effort alone. It is about using the right signals at the right times so the brain receives a clearer message about when to be awake and when to sleep. Light, consistency, and daily habits can all serve as time cues. When used deliberately, they can help move the internal clock earlier, later, or into a steadier pattern that better fits daily life.

That process takes patience. Circadian timing does not usually change overnight, and it does not respond well to abrupt swings. Small, repeated signals are often more powerful than dramatic changes. A stable wake time, morning light, reduced evening light, regular meals, and predictable activity patterns can gradually shape sleep timing in a way that feels more natural than forcing bedtime alone.

It also helps to recognize that not every sleep problem is the same. Someone who naturally falls asleep very late is dealing with a different pattern from someone who becomes sleepy far too early in the evening. Shift work, travel, and irregular schedules create additional forms of disruption. Some patterns are temporary, while others are persistent and biologically driven. Knowing the difference matters, because the strategy should match the pattern.

As you move through the material that follows, the focus will stay on what is practical and specific: how the body clock works, how to notice when it is off, and how to begin guiding it back toward a healthier rhythm. The goal is not perfect sleep every night. The goal is a more reliable rhythm that supports better rest, better alertness, and a daily life that feels less like a fight against time.

Chapter 1: Why Your Body Clock Matters

Before sleep can be improved, it helps to understand that the body is not governed by a single on-off switch. It runs on a coordinated timing system that influences when you feel alert, when you begin to wind down, and how well your body prepares for the next day. When that timing is steady, daily life tends to feel more predictable. When it slips out of alignment, even ordinary routines can start to feel harder than they should. The sections that follow explain the structure behind that timing system and why its signals matter so much for sleep, daytime functioning, and overall health.

How the circadian system works in everyday life

In everyday life, the circadian system acts like a timing layer running underneath everything you do. It does not simply decide whether you are asleep or awake; it helps set the pace for alertness, digestion, temperature, hormone release, and the natural rise and fall of energy across the day. That is why some hours feel naturally easier for focus, exercise, meals, or rest, even before you account for habit or motivation. The body is constantly reading time, and it uses that information to prepare you for what is likely to come next.

One of the clearest ways this shows up is in the daily pattern of sleepiness and alertness. Most people are not equally capable at every hour. There is often a predictable stretch of stronger wakefulness in the morning and early afternoon, followed by a softer dip later in the day, and then a growing drive for sleep in the evening. This pattern is not just a matter of willpower or sleep hygiene. It reflects internal timing signals that influence how sleepy you feel, how easily you concentrate, and how much effort ordinary tasks require. When your schedule matches that rhythm, daily life tends to feel smoother. When it conflicts with it, even simple responsibilities can feel disproportionately hard.

Light is one of the strongest signals shaping that timing. Morning light tells the brain that a new day has begun, helping set the pace for alertness and pushing the internal clock in the direction of earlier wakefulness. Darkness, or reduced light exposure later in the day, supports the transition toward sleep. This is why the timing of light matters so much. Bright evening light can tell the brain to stay active when it should be winding down, while dim, predictable light at night helps preserve the body's expectation that sleep is approaching. In modern life, artificial lighting and screens can blur those signals, making it easier to drift away from the natural day-night pattern.

The circadian system also works through the body's internal chemistry. Hormones and other biological signals rise and fall on a schedule that affects how you feel and function. Cortisol, for example, tends to increase in the morning as part of the normal waking process, while melatonin rises later in the day as part of the transition toward sleep. Core body temperature, digestion, and metabolism also follow timing patterns. These rhythms help explain why appetite, digestion, and energy are often not constant from hour to hour. A late meal may feel different from an early one, and a workout at one time of day may feel easier than at another, even if the effort is the same.

Because the circadian system is tied to so many functions, its influence shows up in ordinary routines. Getting out of bed, starting work, eating breakfast, driving in traffic, attending a meeting, and trying to fall asleep all happen against a background of internal timing. If that timing is aligned, the body provides support at the right moments. If it is shifted, the same activities can feel oddly mismatched. A person may be physically present but mentally foggy in the morning, then unexpectedly alert late at night. Another may feel hungry at times when meals are not convenient, or too sluggish to exercise when the schedule says it should be easy. These are not random inconveniences; they are signs that the timing system is speaking a different language than the calendar.

This is also why consistency matters so much. The circadian system learns from repeated cues. Regular wake times, meal times, light exposure, and activity patterns all reinforce the body's sense of when day begins and ends. When those cues are stable, the system can anticipate what comes next and adjust accordingly. When they change constantly, the body receives mixed messages. Sleeping in late one day, staying up much later the next, eating at widely different times, or spending long stretches in bright light at night can all weaken the clarity of those signals. Over time, that makes it harder for the body to know when to be alert and when to power down.

For people with circadian rhythm sleep problems, this everyday timing system is often the hidden source of the struggle. The issue is not simply that sleep is poor; it is that the body is being asked to sleep, wake, eat, and function at times that do not match its internal schedule. Understanding that mismatch changes how the problem is viewed. It shifts the focus away from trying harder and toward working with timing signals that can be measured, adjusted, and gradually retrained. Once you see how the circadian system operates in ordinary life, the pattern behind symptoms such as late-night alertness, morning exhaustion, or daytime sluggishness becomes easier to recognize and address.

The role of the brain's master clock and peripheral clocks

The brain's master clock sits in a small region of the hypothalamus called the suprachiasmatic nucleus, or SCN. It receives direct information about light from the eyes and uses that input to coordinate daily timing across the body. In practical terms, the SCN helps decide when the body should be in a daytime mode of alertness and when it should shift toward nighttime biology: lower core temperature, rising sleep pressure, changes in hormone release, and a slower metabolic pace. This central clock does not merely respond to sleep; it helps organize the conditions that make sleep and wakefulness easier or harder at specific times.

That master clock is especially important because it is not the only clock in the body. Nearly every organ and tissue contains its own peripheral clock, including the liver, gut, pancreas, muscles, fat tissue, and immune cells. These local clocks help regulate processes such as digestion, blood sugar handling, energy use, and tissue repair. When they are synchronized with the SCN, the body functions with a kind of internal coordination: the brain expects wakefulness, the digestive system is ready to process meals, and muscles and metabolism are prepared for activity. When they drift out of step, the body can feel as if different systems are living on different schedules.

This separation between the master clock and peripheral clocks explains why circadian problems often show up as more than just trouble falling asleep. A person may feel sleepy at the wrong time, but also notice appetite changes, sluggish digestion, afternoon crashes, or a sense that exercise feels harder than usual. The brain may be signaling one time of day while the liver or gut is still operating on another. In that situation, sleep is only one part of the mismatch. The whole system is out of alignment, which is why symptoms can seem broad and inconsistent rather than limited to the bedroom.

Light is the main cue that keeps the master clock anchored, but peripheral clocks are influenced by additional signals, especially meal timing, physical activity, and regular daily routines. This is one reason a person can sometimes feel “off” even when they are getting enough hours in bed. If sleep timing shifts late on weekends, meals become irregular, or activity happens at unpredictable times, the peripheral clocks may begin to follow their own patterns. The SCN still tries to coordinate the system, but the rest of the body may receive mixed messages. Over time, that can make it harder to feel naturally sleepy at night and naturally alert during the day.

The relationship between central and peripheral clocks also helps explain why consistency matters so much in circadian treatment. A single night of earlier sleep or a one-time morning light session can help, but lasting change usually requires repeated signals that teach both the master clock and the body’s local clocks the same time cue. The SCN tends to respond most strongly to light, especially at the right time of day, while peripheral clocks respond more readily to regular patterns of eating, movement, and wakefulness. When those cues are aligned, the body gets a clearer message: this is morning, this is daytime, this is evening, this is night.

Because the clocks in the body are connected but not identical, treatment strategies often work best when they address the whole timing system rather than sleep alone. For example, a person trying to shift earlier may benefit not only from morning light and a fixed wake time, but also from earlier meals and a steady evening wind-down. Those habits do not “force” sleep in a mechanical way. Instead, they reinforce the timing signals that help the brain’s clock and the body’s peripheral clocks settle into the same rhythm. The goal is coordinated timing, not just exhaustion.

It is also useful to remember that the master clock is influential, but it is not inflexible. It can be nudged by repeated exposure to the right cues, and the peripheral clocks can gradually follow. That is why circadian improvement often happens in stages rather than all at once. First, wakefulness may become a little more predictable. Then energy may stabilize. Then sleep may begin to arrive more naturally at the desired hour. These changes reflect a system coming back into alignment, with the brain's master clock leading and the peripheral clocks falling into step behind it.

Why timing affects energy, mood, and metabolism

Timing matters because the body does not manage energy, mood, and metabolism as separate systems. It coordinates them as one daily program. When your internal clock is aligned, the body can anticipate what is coming next: wakefulness in the morning, steady alertness through the day, a gradual shift toward rest at night, and efficient use of fuel in between. When timing is off, the same systems may still function, but they do so at the wrong hour. That mismatch can make a person feel tired yet restless, hungry yet unsatisfied, foggy yet unable to sleep, or emotionally flat even when nothing obvious has changed in life circumstances.

Energy is one of the clearest places this timing shows up. The circadian system helps regulate core body temperature, cortisol release, and the normal rise in alertness that supports getting out of bed and staying engaged during the day. When the clock is set appropriately, the body receives a stronger biological signal for daytime performance and a clearer signal for nighttime recovery. When the clock is delayed, advanced, or repeatedly disrupted, that signal becomes less reliable. A person may wake before the body is ready, push through the morning with effort, and then feel a second wind late at night when sleep should be approaching. From the outside, this can look like poor discipline or inconsistent habits. Biologically, it often reflects a timing problem rather than a lack of willpower.

Mood is closely tied to the same timing network. The brain is not simply more alert or less alert at certain hours; it is also more or less resilient. Sleep timing affects emotional regulation, stress tolerance, and the ability to concentrate without becoming overwhelmed. When circadian rhythms are disrupted, people often notice irritability, anxiety, low motivation, or a sense of being emotionally "off" before they can explain why. Part of this comes from sleep loss itself, but part comes from misalignment between the brain's internal night and the demands of the external day. If the brain is still in a biological evening while work, school, or family responsibilities require daytime functioning, emotional control can feel harder and small frustrations can land with greater force.

Metabolism is equally sensitive to timing. The body handles food differently depending on the time of day, because insulin sensitivity, digestive activity, appetite hormones, and energy storage all follow daily rhythms. In a well-timed system, meals are more likely to be processed efficiently during the active part of the day, when the body is prepared to use incoming energy. When eating drifts late into the night, or when sleep and wake times vary widely, the body may be asked to digest and regulate blood sugar at a biologically inconvenient hour. Over time, that can contribute to heavier feeling after meals, stronger cravings, irregular appetite, and less stable energy. The issue is not that a single late meal causes lasting harm; it is that repeated timing mismatch can gradually push the metabolic system out of its preferred rhythm.

This is one reason circadian disruption can affect weight, blood sugar, and long-term health even when total food intake does not seem dramatically different. The body is not only concerned with how much energy comes in, but also when it arrives. A late schedule can encourage late eating, reduced morning appetite, and a pattern of catching up on calories when the body is biologically less prepared to handle them. At the same time, poor sleep timing can alter hunger signals and make higher-calorie foods more appealing. The result is a feedback loop: misaligned sleep changes eating patterns, and irregular eating can further weaken circadian timing.

The same timing principles help explain why people with circadian rhythm disorders often report feeling “fine” at unusual hours but unable to function when they need to. If your internal night begins too late, then evening may be your most alert period even while the rest of the household is winding down. If your internal morning arrives too early, you may wake before dawn with a clear head and then fade by midafternoon. In both cases, the body is not failing to produce energy; it is producing energy on a schedule that does not match the demands of daily life. That mismatch can make concentration, appetite, and emotional steadiness feel unpredictable from one day to the next.

Understanding this connection changes the way symptoms should be interpreted. A person who feels low, sluggish, or metabolically “off” is not necessarily dealing with separate problems in mood, sleep, and digestion. Those complaints may all be expressions of the same underlying timing disturbance. That is why improving circadian alignment can have broad effects. When sleep becomes more regular and better timed, many people notice not only better rest but also clearer thinking, more stable emotions, and a more natural pattern of hunger and energy across the day. The body responds to timing because timing is one of the main ways it organizes its work.

Common signs that your body clock is misaligned

When the body clock is misaligned, the signs rarely show up as one dramatic symptom. More often, they appear as a pattern: sleep feels hard to start at the expected time, waking feels harder than it should, and the day seems to unfold with an odd mismatch between your energy and the clock on the wall. People often describe this as being "tired but wired," but the experience can be broader than that. You may feel sluggish in the morning, alert late at night, or both within the same 24-hour period. The key clue is not just poor sleep, but sleep and wakefulness that seem to arrive at the wrong times.

One of the most common signs is a consistent delay in sleep onset. If you regularly lie awake for a long time after getting into bed, especially when you are trying to sleep at a socially normal hour, that can signal that your internal timing is still promoting wakefulness. This is different from the occasional restless night. A misaligned clock tends to create a repeatable pattern: you are not simply having trouble sleeping because of stress or a one-off disruption; you are sleepy much later than you want to be. The result is often a cycle of going to bed early, getting frustrated, and then spending more time awake in bed, which can make the mismatch feel even stronger.

On the other end of the day, another sign is difficulty waking at the time you need to rise. The alarm may feel like it is arriving in the middle of biological night rather than at the end of sleep. You may hit snooze repeatedly, feel mentally foggy for a long stretch after waking, or need several cups of coffee before you feel functional. This is especially telling when the problem is most pronounced on school or workdays and less noticeable when you are allowed to follow your own schedule. That difference suggests your sleep timing may be driven more by your internal clock than by your obligations.

Daytime symptoms can be just as revealing. A misaligned circadian rhythm often shows up as predictable dips in alertness at certain hours, especially in the morning, early afternoon, or late evening depending on the direction of the shift. Some people notice that concentration, memory, and decision-making are worse at times when they are expected to perform well. Others feel unusually irritable, emotionally flat, or sensitive to minor stressors. Because timing affects more than sleep, a shifted clock can make the whole day feel uneven: energy may come in waves, with brief bursts of productivity followed by long stretches of fatigue or brain fog.

Changes in appetite and meal timing can also offer clues. If you find yourself hungry very late at night, skipping breakfast without much effort, or craving food at times that do not match your usual routine, that may reflect a clock that is not aligned with the day. The same is true for exercise and social behavior. Some people feel strongest and most motivated late in the evening, then struggle to function in the morning. Others become sleepy unusually early and cannot stay engaged through the evening. These patterns matter because they show that the body is not only misjudging sleep time; it is organizing the rest of its daily rhythms around a different schedule.

It is also useful to notice how your sleep changes across the week. A person with a misaligned clock may sleep reasonably well on free days but fall apart when forced into a conventional schedule. That can look like sleeping in late on weekends, feeling more alert at night, and then dreading the return to early mornings. In some cases, the body seems to "catch up" only after several days off, which can make the problem easy to dismiss as lifestyle-related. But if the pattern repeats even when you are trying to be consistent, it suggests the issue may be biological timing rather than simple bad habits.

Physical signs can point in the same direction. You may notice that your body temperature, hunger, bowel habits, or sense of alertness do not line up neatly with your intended schedule. Some people feel cold and slow in the morning, then suddenly more awake late at night. Others experience a kind of internal jet lag, as if the body is operating in a different time zone from the one they live in. None of these signs alone proves a circadian rhythm disorder, but taken together they can reveal a meaningful pattern. The more regular the mismatch, the more likely it is that the issue involves timing signals rather than random sleep trouble.

The most important thing to watch for is consistency. Anyone can have an occasional late night, a rough morning, or a temporary stretch of poor sleep. Circadian misalignment becomes more likely when the same timing problem keeps returning, when your best sleep happens at hours that do not fit your life, and when your alertness seems to rise and fall according to its own schedule. That pattern is often the first hint that the body clock needs help, and recognizing it early can prevent years of trying to solve a timing problem with willpower alone.

Chapter 2: Recognizing Circadian Rhythm Sleep Disorders

Circadian rhythm sleep disorders are not all the same, and recognizing the pattern matters before any strategy can work well. Some people consistently struggle to fall asleep until very late, while others become sleepy far earlier than the rest of the household. Others live in repeated cycles of changing shifts, crossing time zones, or unpredictable schedules that keep the body from settling into a stable rhythm. In some cases, the pattern is temporary and tied to a specific disruption; in others, it is persistent and reflects an underlying timing mismatch that shows up again and again.

Delayed sleep phase: when sleep comes too late

Delayed sleep phase disorder is more than being a "night owl." Many people prefer late evenings, but in delayed sleep phase, the body's internal timing is shifted so far back that sleep does not feel possible until very late at night or even the early morning hours. The problem is not simply that the person chooses to stay up. The circadian system is sending a late signal for sleep, and the result is a repeated mismatch between when the body wants to rest and when life requires wakefulness. Bedtime may come and go with little sleepiness, while the first hours of the night feel alert, restless, or oddly productive.

This pattern often becomes most visible on school or work days. A person may lie in bed for a long time before falling asleep, then struggle to wake up at a socially normal hour. Mornings can feel heavy and disorienting, with the strongest sleepiness occurring exactly when the day is supposed to begin. By afternoon or evening, energy may improve sharply, creating the impression that the body "finally wakes up" long after everyone else is already winding down. That late shift is a hallmark of the disorder. It is not laziness, lack of discipline, or poor motivation. The timing system itself is delayed.

Delayed sleep phase can be especially confusing because sleep quality is often fairly normal once sleep finally begins. The person may sleep deeply and for a full duration if allowed to follow the delayed schedule. That detail matters. It shows that the issue is usually not an inability to sleep, but an inability to sleep at the desired clock time. A teenager who cannot fall asleep before 2:00 a.m. and then sleeps soundly until late morning, or an adult who naturally drifts toward a 3:00 a.m. bedtime and 11:00 a.m. wake time, may be following a stable but delayed rhythm. The trouble starts when obligations force an earlier rise time and the body has not yet shifted.

Several factors can push the clock later or reinforce a late pattern. Bright light in the evening, especially from screens and indoor lighting, can delay the brain's timing signals. Irregular sleep and wake times can weaken the cues that keep the rhythm anchored. Sleeping in on weekends, taking long late naps, and spending most evenings in low-light indoor environments can all make the body more likely to drift later. In some people, the tendency appears to have a stronger biological basis, which is why the pattern can persist even when the person is trying hard to "go to bed earlier." The effort may be sincere, but effort alone does not always overcome a shifted circadian phase.

One useful way to think about delayed sleep phase is to separate sleep drive from circadian timing. Sleep drive builds the longer you stay awake, so someone with this disorder may eventually become exhausted enough to fall asleep very late. But the circadian system is still resisting sleep earlier in the evening. That is why going to bed at 10:30 p.m. may lead to prolonged wakefulness, frustration, and clock-watching rather than rest. The person is trying to sleep at a biological time that still feels like evening alertness. When that happens night after night, the bed itself can become associated with effort and disappointment, which adds another layer of difficulty.

The disorder often shows up in daily life as a cycle of late sleep, hard mornings, and compensatory behavior. A person may depend on alarms, caffeine, or repeated snoozing to get through the first part of the day. They may feel more themselves in the late afternoon and evening, then promise to correct the schedule the next night, only to find that sleep again refuses to arrive early. Over time, this can affect school attendance, work performance, mood, and family routines. It may also create tension with others who interpret the pattern as a choice rather than a timing problem. That misunderstanding can be painful, especially when the person is already trying to function against the grain of their own biology.

Recognizing delayed sleep phase means noticing the pattern, not just the bedtime. The key clues are consistent late sleep onset, difficulty waking at conventional hours, and a tendency for alertness to improve late in the day. If the schedule is allowed to run on its own, sleep may be adequate but shifted. If the schedule is forced earlier, sleep often becomes shorter and more fragmented because the body is not yet ready. Once that pattern is identified, the next question is not how to "try harder" to sleep early, but how to send stronger and more consistent timing signals so the clock can begin moving in the right direction.

Advanced sleep phase: when sleep comes too early

Advanced sleep phase disorder is the opposite of delayed sleep phase in one important way: the internal clock is shifted earlier than the schedule most people need to follow. Sleepiness arrives too soon in the evening, often long before the person wants to go to bed, and waking comes too early in the morning, sometimes after only a few hours of sleep. The result can look, from the outside, like someone who simply likes early nights and early mornings. In reality, the timing is often rigid and biologically driven. The person may not be choosing to get sleepy at 7:30 p.m. or waking at 3:30 a.m.; the body is sending those signals on its own schedule.

This pattern can be easy to miss because it may seem socially acceptable, even admirable, to go to bed early. But the key question is not whether the bedtime is early. It is whether the timing matches the person's life and whether sleep is actually restorative. Someone with advanced sleep phase may fall asleep quickly in the early evening, sleep soundly for a while, and then wake before dawn feeling fully alert, with no ability to return to sleep. By midmorning, that same person may already feel as if the day is long, while the evening brings a repeated wave of sleepiness that is hard to resist. The clock is not just early; it is compressed.

Because the wake time is so early, advanced sleep phase can create a different kind of daytime problem than people expect. The person may be technically getting enough hours on paper, but the timing still leaves them out of sync with work, family, or social life. Evening activities become difficult to sustain, and the early morning awakening may happen at an hour that prevents a full night's rest. If the person gives in to the early sleepiness every night, they may go to bed before they are actually ready, which can reinforce the pattern. If they fight it and stay up later, they may become sleep deprived, which adds another layer of fatigue on top of the circadian shift.

Advanced sleep phase tends to be especially noticeable when the person's schedule requires evening alertness. A dinner that stretches later than usual, a family event, a class, or a work obligation can feel disproportionately hard to manage because the body is already leaning hard toward sleep. At the same time, the early morning wake-up can be frustratingly consistent. The person may set an alarm for 6:00 a.m. and still wake at 4:00 a.m. with the same level of alertness, as if the body has decided that the night is over. This is one reason the disorder can be mistaken for simple aging, personality, or habit. Early rising is common in older adults, but advanced sleep phase is more than a preference for early hours; it is a stable timing shift that can interfere with functioning.

Light exposure plays a central role in why this pattern develops and how it can be managed. In advanced sleep phase, the clock is often running too early, so evening light can be helpful because it provides a signal that delays the body's timing slightly. That does not mean bright light late at night is automatically good for everyone, or that the goal is to stay up under harsh lighting for hours. The timing and amount matter. But compared with delayed sleep phase, where morning light is used to move the clock earlier, advanced sleep phase often calls for the opposite strategy: protecting the evening from becoming too dark too soon, while avoiding overly early morning light that can push the clock even earlier.

Daily habits can either support or worsen the pattern. If a person with advanced sleep phase consistently goes to bed the moment sleepiness appears, the body may learn that very early evening is the correct sleep signal. If they wake at dawn and immediately expose themselves to bright morning light, the early timing can become even more entrenched. On the other hand, extending wakefulness into the evening with meaningful activity, moderate light, and a predictable routine may help hold the clock later. The point is not to force the body into artificial alertness for its own sake. It is to create a stable, repeatable set of cues that tell the circadian system that evening still belongs to the waking day.

It is also important to separate advanced sleep phase from ordinary early rising caused by short sleep, stress, or a temporarily busy schedule. Someone who is exhausted may fall asleep early because they are overextended, not because their circadian clock is advanced. Someone under stress may wake early with racing thoughts rather than with true biological alertness. In advanced sleep phase, the pattern is more regular than that. Sleep comes early even when the person is not especially sleep deprived, and waking comes early even when there is a clear desire to sleep longer. The consistency of the pattern is one of the strongest clues that the issue is circadian rather than simply behavioral.

For many people, the hardest part is accepting that an early bedtime is not always a healthy bedtime. If sleep is arriving too soon, the goal is not to celebrate the early hour, but to ask whether the timing is stealing rest from the end of the night and leaving the person misaligned with the rest of life. That distinction matters because it changes the strategy. Instead of treating the early sleepiness as a fixed personality trait, the next step is to look at how light, routine, and wake timing may be helping lock the clock into an earlier position than the person needs.

Shift work and rotating schedules

Shift work creates one of the clearest examples of circadian misalignment because it asks the body to perform daytime functions at night and nighttime functions during the day. The problem is not just shortened sleep. It is the repeated demand to sleep, eat, and stay alert at hours when the body clock is sending the opposite message. A person may finish a night shift feeling exhausted but unable to fall asleep right away, then wake too early because of light, noise, or family obligations. Even if total sleep time is partly recovered, the timing is often fragmented enough that the internal clock never fully settles.

Rotating schedules can be even harder than a stable night shift because the body is forced to keep changing direction. Just as the circadian system begins to adapt, the next schedule change pulls it somewhere else. Forward rotation, such as day to evening to night, is generally easier to tolerate than backward rotation, but either pattern can leave a person feeling chronically off balance. The issue is not simply that sleep is shorter on some days. The deeper problem is that the brain and body cannot predict when to prepare for wakefulness, digestion, temperature changes, and sleep. That uncertainty makes it harder to build a reliable rhythm.

People working nights often notice a familiar pattern: the first part of the shift may feel manageable, then alertness drops in the early morning hours, and after work the body becomes strangely awake again. This is partly because the circadian system has its own daily wave of alertness and sleepiness, and that wave does not automatically move just because the schedule has changed. Light exposure at the wrong time can reinforce the mismatch. Bright light during the commute home can signal daytime to the brain, making it harder to sleep after the shift. Conversely, darkness during the work period can make alertness harder to maintain, especially in the lowest circadian hours before dawn.

Because of that, managing shift work is less about forcing the body to behave like a daytime sleeper and more about creating a controlled set of signals that reduce conflict. The goal is to protect sleep during the sleep window and support alertness during the work window. For many people, that means using light strategically, limiting bright light on the way home, and making the sleep environment as dark and quiet as possible. Blackout curtains, eye masks, earplugs, white noise, and a cool room can all help the body read the post-shift period as a legitimate time for rest. If sleep is repeatedly interrupted by family responsibilities or daytime noise, the body receives mixed messages that make adaptation much harder.

Meal timing also matters more than many shift workers expect. Eating a large meal in the biological night can send signals to peripheral clocks that conflict with the brain's timing system. That does not mean a night worker must eat perfectly on a textbook schedule, but it does mean that heavy, irregular, or constant eating can add another layer of confusion. Smaller meals during the shift, with the largest meal placed closer to the main waking period when possible, may feel easier on digestion and energy. Caffeine can be useful early in a shift, but if it extends too far into the night, it can delay sleep long after the work is over.

Rotating schedules often require a different mindset from fixed night work because the body is asked to remain flexible rather than fully adapt. In those cases, the best strategy is often to anchor the sleep pattern as much as possible around the most stable part of the week. A consistent wake time on non-work days, or at least a limited range of wake times, can reduce the amount of resetting the body has to do. Long weekend sleep-ins may feel restorative in the moment, but they can deepen the sense of jet lag when the next work block begins. The body clock responds to repetition, not to occasional recovery sleep alone.

It also helps to distinguish between coping and adapting. Coping means getting through the schedule with enough sleep and alertness to function safely. Adapting means shifting the circadian system enough that the schedule feels more natural. Not every shift worker can or should try to fully adapt, especially if the schedule changes frequently. In many cases, partial adaptation is the realistic target. That may include using light at specific times, protecting a dark sleep period, and keeping social and family commitments from erasing the sleep opportunity. The more predictable the pattern around the work shift, the more the body can learn what to expect, even if the clock itself never becomes fully aligned.

When shift work is unavoidable, safety deserves special attention. Drowsiness during a commute, slowed reaction time on the job, and frequent unplanned naps are signs that the schedule is exceeding the body's current capacity to compensate. Those signals should not be ignored or treated as weakness. They are often evidence that the circadian system is being asked to perform under conditions it was not designed for. In that situation, the most effective improvements usually come from reducing light and schedule chaos, protecting the main sleep episode, and using timing deliberately rather than trying to rely on willpower alone.

Jet lag and temporary clock disruption

Jet lag is a temporary circadian mismatch caused by rapid travel across time zones. The body clock does not reset the moment the plane lands. Instead, it continues to run on the timing it learned from the departure location, while the destination demands a different schedule for sleep, meals, light exposure, and alertness. That is why a traveler can arrive physically exhausted yet still lie awake at the "wrong" local bedtime, or wake up in the middle of the night feeling as if it is morning back home. The problem is not simply lost sleep from the trip itself. It is a short-term disagreement between internal time and external time.

The size and direction of the time change matter. Crossing one or two time zones may create mild grogginess, but larger shifts can produce several days of uneven sleep, digestive changes, reduced concentration, and a sense that the day is unfolding at the wrong pace. Eastward travel usually feels harder because it requires the body to fall asleep and wake earlier than it prefers. Westward travel often feels easier because it allows a later bedtime and later wake time, which is closer to the natural tendency of many internal clocks. Even so, either direction can disrupt sleep if the schedule is packed, the hotel room is bright or noisy, or the traveler keeps irregular hours after arrival.

Temporary clock disruption is not limited to airplanes and time zones. Any abrupt change in routine can shake the timing system enough to cause short-lived misalignment. A late-night event, a string of early morning obligations, an overnight drive, a sudden change in work hours, or several days of poor sleep can all create a similar pattern: the body wants one timing schedule while life demands another. In these cases, the circadian system is not permanently disordered, but it is temporarily off balance. That distinction matters because the body usually knows how to realign if given stable cues and enough time.

What makes jet lag especially noticeable is that it affects more than sleepiness. The clock that governs alertness is also tied to digestion, body temperature, and the timing of hormones that help organize the day. A traveler may notice that meals feel too early or too late, appetite is irregular, or energy rises and falls at strange times. Some people feel foggy in the morning, wired in the evening, and then unexpectedly sleepy in the middle of the day. Others become irritable or get headaches. These symptoms can be easy to blame on stress or travel fatigue alone, but the timing pattern often reveals the true cause: the body is still living in the old time zone.

Recovery depends on giving the circadian system clear signals about the new local time. Light is usually the strongest cue. Bright outdoor light in the morning helps tell the brain that the day has started, while reducing bright light late at night helps prevent the clock from drifting later. Meals, movement, and wake time also matter because they reinforce the message that local daytime is the new reference point. A traveler who sleeps in, naps for long stretches, eats at odd times, and spends the evening in bright light may prolong the mismatch. A traveler who gets up at a consistent local wake time, seeks daylight soon after rising, and keeps evening light low usually adapts more quickly.

It can help to think in terms of direction rather than simply "getting over" jet lag. After eastward travel, the goal is often to shift earlier, which means using morning light and protecting the evening from excess brightness. After westward travel, the body usually needs to shift later, which can make late afternoon and evening light more useful while still avoiding a pattern of sleeping too late the next morning. The exact approach depends on the number of time zones crossed, the timing of arrival, and how quickly the person must function on local time. A short trip may not justify a full adjustment, but a longer stay usually does.

Temporary disruption also improves when expectations are realistic. The first day after travel is often not a fair test of a person's normal sleep ability. A poor night in a hotel, a red-eye flight, or a schedule that forces early meetings can make anyone feel off. The key question is whether the problem resolves as the body receives stable timing cues. If sleep remains difficult only for a few days after travel and then settles, that pattern fits temporary clock disruption. If the same misalignment keeps returning without travel, or if the person never seems to adapt even after several days in one time zone, it may point to a deeper circadian issue that deserves closer attention.

When irregular patterns signal a deeper problem

Not every irregular sleep pattern is a circadian rhythm disorder, and that distinction matters. Many people have weeks or months where sleep is inconsistent because of stress, illness, parenting demands, travel, pain, shift changes, or a demanding schedule. In those situations, the body clock may be strained, but it is not necessarily broken. The question is whether the pattern is temporary and explainable, or whether it keeps returning in the same way even when life is relatively stable.

A deeper problem becomes more likely when the timing of sleep seems to follow a stubborn internal pattern rather than the demands of the day. For example, you may feel alert until very late night after night, no matter how tired you are, or you may become sleepy so early that staying awake for normal evening activities feels like a struggle. You may also notice that weekends, vacations, or time off do not fully normalize your sleep. If you can sleep "fine" only when allowed to follow your preferred schedule, but that schedule is incompatible with work, school, or family life, the issue may be more than a bad habit. It may be a timing disorder that is repeatedly pulling sleep toward a fixed late or early window.

Another warning sign is consistency. Ordinary sleep disruption often changes shape from one week to the next. Circadian rhythm disorders tend to be more repeatable. The person falls asleep at nearly the same late hour, wakes at nearly the same early hour, or becomes sleepy at a predictable time each day, even when trying hard to adjust. This regularity can be easy to miss because the pattern may look like discipline, personality, or preference from the outside. But when the body keeps producing the same timing problem over and over, it suggests that the internal clock is driving the behavior more strongly than choice alone.

It is also important to notice what happens when you try to shift the schedule. If you go to bed earlier, do you lie awake for a long time with no sign of sleepiness? If you try to sleep later, do you wake up anyway, almost as if an alarm went off inside your body? These reactions can point to a clock that is anchored at the wrong time. In a circadian disorder, the problem is not simply that sleep is too short. The problem is that the sleep drive and the body's timing signals are arriving out of phase with the clock on the wall. That mismatch can make the person feel as though sleep is being forced rather than naturally allowed.

Daytime symptoms can provide additional clues. When circadian timing is off, the consequences often spill beyond bedtime. You may feel unusually foggy in the morning, more alert at night than seems reasonable, or sharply tired at a specific point each afternoon. Mood may also follow the timing pattern, with irritability, low motivation, or a sense of being mentally "off" at certain hours. Some people notice that appetite, digestion, and concentration shift in parallel with their sleep timing. These broader effects matter because they suggest the issue is not only about getting enough hours in bed. It is about when the body expects to be awake, asleep, and metabolically active.

At the same time, not every unusual pattern means a circadian disorder. Short sleep from chronic overwork, anxiety-driven insomnia, depression, medication effects, substance use, untreated pain, snoring-related breathing problems, or restless legs can all create irregular sleep. In those cases, the timing may look chaotic because something else is interfering with sleep itself. That is why it helps to ask a simple question: is the main problem that sleep is unavailable, or that sleep is available at the wrong time? Circadian disorders are defined by timing. Other conditions may disturb sleep for different reasons, even when the end result feels similar.

When the pattern is persistent, repeatable, and tied to a clear mismatch between your sleep timing and your required schedule, it deserves closer attention. That is especially true if the problem is affecting work, school, safety, relationships, or mental health. A person who regularly cannot fall asleep until 2 or 3 a.m., or who repeatedly wakes at 4 or 5 a.m. despite trying to shift, is not simply being inconsistent. The body may be telling a very specific timing story.

Recognizing that story is the first step toward choosing the right kind of intervention instead of just trying harder to sleep on command.

Chapter 3: Finding Your Personal Sleep Pattern

Before any adjustment can work, you need a clearer picture of what your sleep is already doing on its own. Many people try to force a schedule into place without first noticing the rhythm their body is actually following, and that often leads to frustration because the problem is treated as a lack of discipline rather than a timing pattern. The goal here is not to judge your habits or to build a perfect record overnight. It is to gather enough information to see when sleep tends to arrive, when alertness tends to rise, and what seems to shift those patterns from day to day.

Building a simple sleep and energy log

A simple sleep and energy log is one of the most useful tools for finding out what your body clock is actually doing. It does not need to be elaborate, and it should not feel like homework you can never keep up with. The purpose is to capture enough information to reveal patterns that are easy to miss in the moment: when you naturally get sleepy, when you wake without an alarm, how alert or foggy you feel at different times of day, and what seems to push your rhythm earlier or later. A good log turns vague impressions into something you can observe over time.

Start with the basics: bedtime, estimated time to fall asleep, number of awakenings, wake time, and whether you used an alarm. Then add a simple rating for how you felt on waking and another for your energy at a few points during the day. You do not need a detailed report every hour. Three or four check-ins are enough for most people. For example, you might rate morning energy, midafternoon energy, evening alertness, and overall sleep quality on a scale from 1 to 5. The goal is consistency, not precision down to the minute. If you can keep the format simple, you are more likely to keep using it long enough to see a pattern.

It also helps to record the timing of a few key cues that influence circadian rhythm. Light exposure matters, so note whether you got outdoor light soon after waking, spent much of the day indoors, or used bright light late at night. Meals matter too, especially the timing of breakfast, dinner, and late snacks. Exercise, caffeine, alcohol, naps, and unusually stressful events can all affect sleep timing and quality, so mark those when they are relevant. You do not need to document every detail of your day. Just note the events that might reasonably have shifted your alertness or sleep drive.

Keep the language in the log plain and factual. Instead of writing "I slept badly," try "went to bed at 12:45 a.m., fell asleep around 2:00 a.m., woke at 6:30 a.m. with alarm, energy 2/5 until noon." That kind of entry is more useful because it separates behavior from interpretation. It also helps you notice whether the issue is sleep timing, sleep duration, sleep fragmentation, or some combination of all three. Over several days, the difference between "I feel tired" and "I fall asleep late, wake early, and crash at 3 p.m." becomes much easier to see.

One of the most important habits is to record your natural sleep window whenever possible. If you wake before an alarm on days off, note the time carefully. If you start feeling sleepy at the same hour most evenings, write that down too. These details can point to your biological timing rather than your scheduled timing. A person who can fall asleep easily at 10:30 p.m. on vacation but not on work nights may be revealing a mismatch between habit and obligation. Another person who gets sleepy at 8:00 p.m. and wakes at 4:30 a.m. even after a full night's sleep may be showing an advanced pattern rather than simple morning preference.

Try to collect enough data to cover both ordinary days and unusual ones. A log that only reflects your best nights or worst nights can be misleading. Three to four weeks is often enough to reveal a stable pattern, especially if your schedule is fairly regular. If your routine changes from day to day, the record may need to be longer. The point is not to prove that every day is identical. It is to see whether your sleep and energy follow a repeatable rhythm even when the details vary. That repeatability is often the clue that biology is driving the pattern.

To make the log manageable, use a format you can complete in under two minutes. Some people prefer a notebook by the bed. Others use a note app or a printed table. Either is fine as long as you can use it consistently. If you miss a day, do not backfill from memory unless you are certain of the details. A few imperfect entries are better than abandoning the log because it feels too demanding. What matters most is creating a record that shows how your sleep and energy move across time, not producing a perfect diary.

As the entries build, look for simple relationships. Do later bedtimes reliably follow late screen use or evening work? Does morning light seem to improve daytime alertness? Do weekend sleep-ins make Monday nights harder? Does a late lunch or evening caffeine push sleep later? These patterns are often more revealing than any single night of poor sleep. A simple log gives you a way to test whether a suspected trigger is actually part of the problem and whether a change in routine is helping your body clock move in the direction you want.

Identifying your natural sleep window

To identify your natural sleep window, begin with the assumption that your body already has a preferred timing pattern, even if that pattern is not the one you want. The goal is not to force sleep earlier or later right away, but to notice when sleep starts to feel possible without a fight. That window is usually easier to detect when you stop treating bedtime as a fixed command and instead observe the point at which sleepiness becomes genuine, steady, and hard to resist. For some people, that happens earlier in the evening than expected. For others, it does not arrive until long after the household has gone quiet. Either way, the pattern is useful because it reflects what the internal clock is doing before outside demands interfere.

A natural sleep window is not the same thing as the time you go to bed, the time you turn off the lights, or the time you finally fall asleep after scrolling, reading, or lying awake. It is the period when your brain and body are most ready to transition into sleep if the conditions are reasonable. You may notice that on some nights you feel a clear drop in alertness, a heavier eyelid sensation, slower thinking, or a strong urge to stop doing anything demanding. That is often the beginning of the window. If you miss it and stay active for another hour or two, sleep may become harder again, not easier, because the body can shift into a second wind. People often mistake that second wind for being "not tired enough," when in fact it is a timing signal that has been passed.

One of the most helpful clues comes from days when you are free of alarms, obligations, and social pressure. On those days, observe when you naturally wake and when you naturally become sleepy at night. If you repeatedly wake at roughly the same time without forcing yourself, that can reveal one edge of your rhythm. If you also notice that sleepiness reliably arrives at a similar clock time, that gives you the other edge. Together, those points help define the sleep window. This is especially important for people who assume they are simply bad sleepers because they cannot fall asleep at a "normal" bedtime. In many cases, the body is not resisting sleep in general; it is resisting sleep at the wrong hour.

It helps to distinguish true sleepiness from fatigue, boredom, or exhaustion. Fatigue can make you feel drained, but still mentally alert or emotionally keyed up. True sleepiness usually brings a softer, more unmistakable shift: you may blink more, lose your train of thought, reread the same sentence, or stop caring about tasks that felt urgent an hour earlier. If your eyes feel heavy but your mind is racing, that can mean the sleep window is approaching but your system is still being stimulated by light, stress, caffeine, or activity. If you feel worn out but cannot imagine sleeping, the problem may be that your body is tired in a general sense while your circadian timing is still sending a wake signal.

Pay attention to consistency across several days rather than trying to judge one night at a time. A single late bedtime after an unusually busy day does not define your rhythm. A natural sleep window shows up as a pattern. You may notice that on quiet evenings you become drowsy at almost the same hour, or that when you sleep without an alarm your wake time clusters within a fairly narrow range. You may also find that your sleep window shifts on weekends, after late-night light exposure, or during periods of stress. Those shifts matter because they show what nudges your clock earlier or later. The more stable the pattern, the more likely it reflects biology rather than habit alone.

When you are trying to locate the window, avoid making the experiment too complicated. Keep your evenings as ordinary as possible while you observe. Write down the time you first feel sleepy, the time you actually go to bed, how long it takes to fall asleep, and whether you wake feeling refreshed or still foggy. If you are consistently sleepy much later than your target bedtime, that suggests your window may be delayed. If you are falling asleep far earlier than desired and waking too early, the window may be advanced. If the timing swings widely from day to day, the issue may be less about a fixed phase disorder and more about inconsistent cues that keep the body clock from settling.

Once you have a sense of the window, the next step is to respect it rather than argue with it. That does not mean surrendering to it permanently. It means using the information to choose smarter timing for change. If your natural sleepiness is arriving at 1:00 a.m., asking your body to sleep at 10:00 p.m. is usually too large a leap. If your window is earlier than you want, staying up much later every night may only deepen the mismatch. In both cases, the starting point is the same: identify the timing your body is already choosing, because that is the baseline from which a realistic reset can begin.

Spotting triggers that push your clock later or earlier

Once you have a sense of your natural sleep window, the next question is what seems to move it. Many people assume their timing is fixed, when in fact it is being nudged day after day by a small set of signals. Some of those signals push the clock later, making sleep drift toward midnight, 1 a.m., or beyond. Others pull it earlier, making evening sleepiness arrive too soon and shortening the usable part of the day. The important point is not whether one trigger acts alone, but whether several triggers are pointing in the same direction and reinforcing the pattern.

Light is usually the strongest trigger, but it is far from the only one. Evening brightness from overhead lights, bright television screens, tablets, phones, and laptops can all delay the brain's nighttime signal. Even if the light does not seem intense, the timing matters. Exposure late in the evening tells the circadian system that day is still going on, which can suppress the rise in sleepiness and make the body feel more alert than it should. For people who already lean late, this effect can be enough to keep bedtime sliding later and later, especially when the evening is quiet and the mind is finally free to engage.

There are also behavioral triggers that can push the clock later without being obvious. Irregular bedtimes are one of the most common. If you stay up late on some nights and go to bed earlier on others, the body may stop learning a reliable pattern and begin to delay in response to the later nights. Long naps, especially late in the afternoon, can reduce the sleep pressure that would normally help you fall asleep at night. Alcohol can also make sleep timing look more settled than it really is, because it may create early drowsiness while fragmenting sleep later in the night. Caffeine is another frequent contributor, particularly when it is used to compensate for poor sleep and then consumed too late in the day to wear off before bedtime.

Stress and mental activation can act like timing triggers as well. A person may not be exposed to much light at night and still find that sleep keeps moving later because the evening has become the only time for work, problem-solving, scrolling, gaming, or emotionally charged conversations. The brain begins to associate that period with alertness rather than rest. Over time, the body may treat late evening as a productive or stimulating part of the day, and sleep becomes harder to initiate even when exhaustion is present. This is one reason the same person can feel sleepy on the couch at 9 p.m. but suddenly wake up once they get into bed and expect sleep to happen.

Triggers that push the clock earlier are less common in everyday life but just as important to notice. Early morning bright light can advance the clock, especially if it is combined with a very early wake time that repeats every day. If you are waking before dawn, commuting in bright light, or spending time outside shortly after rising, your brain may receive a strong signal to shift timing earlier. That can be helpful for some people, but for others it can make evenings feel prematurely sleepy and mornings overly rigid. The same is true for consistently early meals, early exercise, and very early social or work schedules, all of which can reinforce an earlier phase when they happen at the same time each day.

Age and biology can also tilt the timing in an earlier direction. Some people naturally become more morning-oriented as they get older, and that shift may be more noticeable if they are already sensitive to light and routine. Medical conditions, medications, and mood changes can further influence timing. For example, certain sedating medications may make evenings come on too strongly, while depression or chronic fatigue can make the day feel compressed and lead to earlier sleep onset. If sleep is arriving earlier than desired, it is worth considering whether the pattern reflects a true advance of the body clock or a broader issue that is making you feel depleted before night has really begun.

The most useful way to identify triggers is to look for repetition. A single late night does not mean your clock has shifted. A pattern does. Ask what changed on the days when sleep moved later or earlier. Was there more evening light than usual? A missed meal? A long nap? A stressful conversation? An unusually early wake time? A weekend schedule that differed sharply from the workweek? When you compare these details against your sleep log, the same few influences often show up again and again. The goal is not to blame yourself for every late night or early morning, but to separate a random bad night from a signal that is repeatedly steering your rhythm in one direction.

It can help to sort triggers into two groups: those you can change and those you need to work around. You may not be able to control a shift schedule, caregiving demands, or sunrise time, but you can notice how those factors affect your clock and then reduce the impact of the ones within reach. That might mean dimming lights earlier, moving caffeine to the morning, shortening naps, keeping weekend wake times closer to weekday wake times, or creating a more predictable evening routine. The point is to identify the forces that are quietly training your clock so you can decide which ones deserve the most attention.

Using patterns to distinguish habit from biology

One of the most useful things you can do at this stage is stop asking only, "Why am I sleeping this way?" and start asking, "What pattern is this sleep following?" That shift matters because a repeated pattern can reveal whether you are looking at a true circadian tendency, a learned habit, or a mix of both. Habit and biology often look similar from the outside. A person who falls asleep at 1:30 a.m. every night may seem to be choosing a late schedule, but the pattern may actually reflect a delayed body clock, reinforced over time by evening light, stimulating activities, and sleeping in. Another person may appear to be an early sleeper, but the real driver may be exhaustion, low light exposure, or an overly quiet routine that makes the evening collapse happen long before the body's natural sleep window.

The easiest way to separate these influences is to look for consistency across different conditions. If your sleep timing stays almost the same on workdays, weekends, vacations, and low-stress periods, biology is probably playing a stronger role. If your sleep shifts dramatically depending on what you do, when you eat, how much light you get, or whether you stay up with other people, habit is likely contributing more. Most real-life cases are not either-or. The body clock sets a range, and daily behavior can push sleep within that range or even distort it over time. That is why it helps to think in terms of tendencies rather than absolutes. A habit may not create the pattern from nothing, but it can strengthen it until it feels like your personality.

Pay close attention to what happens when external pressure is removed. On days when you do not have to wake to an alarm, do you sleep much later than you intended? Do you naturally feel sleepy at the same late hour even when you try to stay up? Do you wake feeling fully alert at a time that seems too early or too late for your schedule? These details can be more revealing than the bedtime you aim for. For example, someone who goes to bed at 10:30 p.m. because they are trying to be disciplined, but who lies awake for an hour most nights, may be forcing a habit that does not match the underlying clock. In that case, the problem is not a lack of willpower. It is a mismatch between chosen timing and biological timing.

It also helps to notice whether the pattern is stable in one direction. Biology tends to show a repeated pull. A delayed clock usually keeps pushing sleep later, even after several "early" nights, while an advanced clock keeps bringing sleepiness forward, even when the person tries to stay up. Habit, by contrast, often changes more easily when the environment changes. If a late pattern improves noticeably during a week of morning light, steady wake time, and reduced evening stimulation, that suggests the clock is responsive rather than fixed. If nothing changes at all, or the pattern snaps back as soon as structure loosens, the biological component may be stronger than it first appeared.

Another clue is the difference between sleepiness and opportunity. Many people confuse the two. You may have the opportunity to go to bed at a certain hour, but that does not mean your brain is ready for sleep. If you routinely get into bed because the clock says it is time, yet you feel mentally active, physically restless, or oddly alert, the issue may be timing rather than behavior. On the other hand, if you feel sleepy only after a long stretch of evening scrolling, snacking, or television, the sleepiness may be partly self-created by routine and overstimulation. In both cases, the pattern matters more than the isolated night.

Look for the clues that come from the body itself, not just from circumstances. Do you get a predictable "second wind" at night? Do you feel unusually awake after sunset but sluggish in the morning? Do you become sleepy at about the same hour regardless of whether the day was busy or calm? Biological rhythms often show this kind of internal clockwork. Habit usually depends more on cues from the environment and can be altered more quickly by changing those cues. If your sleep pattern persists even when you try to behave differently, that persistence is meaningful. It suggests that your schedule is not simply a product of preference or poor discipline, but of a timing system that has settled into a particular rhythm.

The goal is not to label every pattern as either "all habit" or "all biology." The more useful question is which influence is leading and which is following. A late bedtime may begin as a habit, then become a biological pattern through repetition. A biological tendency may begin as a mild preference, then get amplified by routines that keep reinforcing it. When you start reading your sleep this way, you can stop fighting the wrong battle. Instead of blaming yourself for a pattern that may have a real circadian basis, you can focus on the parts that are adjustable: light, timing, consistency, and the cues that teach the clock what hour it is supposed to be.

Chapter 4: The Science of Resetting the Clock

Resetting the body clock is not a matter of forcing sleep into place; it is a process of giving the brain repeated, reliable information about what time it is. Once you understand that circadian timing responds to signals rather than willpower, the next question becomes which signals matter most and how they work together. Some cues are powerful because they speak directly to the brain's timing center, while others matter because they reinforce the same message day after day until the body begins to expect it. This is where small choices start to matter in a biological way, not just a behavioral one.

How light resets the brain's timing signals

Light is the strongest timing signal the brain receives from the environment. It does not just help you see; it tells the circadian system what part of the day it is and helps set the pace of the internal clock. That message begins at the eyes, where specialized light-sensitive cells detect brightness and send information along a direct pathway to the brain's master clock. This is why light can shift sleep timing so powerfully even when you are not consciously paying attention to it. The brain is always interpreting the light environment, and it uses that information to decide whether to move the body toward daytime alertness or nighttime readiness.

The timing effect of light depends on when it arrives, not simply how bright it is. Morning light tends to push the clock earlier, helping the body prepare for earlier sleep and earlier waking. Light in the evening and at night tends to push the clock later, delaying the internal signal for sleep and making it harder to feel naturally sleepy at a socially expected bedtime. This is one reason a person with delayed sleep phase can feel especially alert late at night: the brain has been receiving a repeated "stay on daytime schedule" message from evening light, whether from indoor lighting, screens, or a bright environment that extends too far into the night.

The brain's response to light is also shaped by the concept of phase shifting. A phase shift is a change in the timing of the circadian clock. When light is delivered at the right time, it can move the clock earlier or later. When it is delivered at the wrong time, it can work against the schedule you are trying to build. That is why light treatment is not just about "getting more light" or "avoiding screens." It is about using light as a timed signal. The same light that helps one person wake up and stabilize a morning routine may be the very thing that keeps another person stuck in a late pattern.

The brain is especially sensitive to light at the edges of the sleep period. Light soon after waking is generally a strong cue that the day has begun, and it helps anchor alertness, body temperature, and hormonal rhythms to the morning. Light late in the evening has the opposite effect, particularly when the body is already preparing for sleep. In practical terms, this means that a bright walk outside after waking can be biologically very different from a bright room late at night, even if both feel like ordinary exposure to light. The clock is reading the timing of the signal, not just the signal itself.

Consistency matters because the circadian system learns from repeated patterns. A single bright morning may help, but a steady morning light routine teaches the brain that wake time is reliable. A single late-night screen session may not derail everything, but repeated evening light exposure can keep reinforcing a later schedule. The clock is not reset by one dramatic event so much as by a pattern of signals that arrive at the same time each day. This is why circadian change often feels gradual. The brain is not being forced into a new rhythm; it is being persuaded by repeated evidence.

Light also interacts with sleep pressure, which is the growing need for sleep that builds across the day. When light is timed well, it helps align sleep pressure with the circadian signal for rest. When light is timed poorly, it can create a mismatch: the body may have enough sleep pressure to feel tired, but the clock is still sending a wakefulness signal. That is when people often describe feeling exhausted yet unable to fall asleep, or sleepy in the wrong part of the day and unexpectedly alert at night. In circadian disorders, that mismatch is often the core problem, and light is one of the main ways to reduce it.

This is also why different people need different light strategies. Someone who naturally falls asleep too late usually needs strong morning light and reduced evening light to move the clock earlier. Someone who becomes sleepy too early may need the opposite pattern, with carefully timed evening light to keep the clock from advancing too far. Shift workers and frequent travelers may need light timing that changes from one day to the next, depending on whether the goal is to stay aligned with a work schedule or adapt to a new time zone. The principle is the same in every case: light is a biological instruction, and the instruction only helps when it matches the timing goal.

Because the brain is reading light as a timing cue, even small changes in the daily light environment can matter more than people expect. Opening the blinds soon after waking, spending time outdoors in the morning, dimming lights in the evening, and limiting bright light close to bedtime all help shape the signal the clock receives. The goal is not perfection. It is to make the light pattern more consistent with the sleep pattern you want the body to learn. Over time, that consistency gives the brain a clearer message about when to be alert, when to slow down, and when to prepare for sleep.

Why consistency beats intensity in circadian change

Circadian change works best when the body receives the same message over and over again. The system that governs sleep timing is highly responsive, but it is not especially impressed by one dramatic effort. A single late-night blackout curtain, one perfect morning light session, or an occasional "reset day" may feel decisive in the moment, yet the clock is built to track patterns, not isolated events. What matters most is whether the signals you send are stable enough for the brain to treat them as reliable time cues.

This is why consistency usually beats intensity. A modest light exposure at the same time each morning can do more for your sleep timing than an occasional extreme effort that is hard to repeat. The circadian system learns from repetition. When wake time, light exposure, meals, and bedtime preparation happen at similar hours, the body begins to predict what comes next. That prediction is what allows the clock to shift and then hold its new position. By contrast, intense but irregular efforts can create a kind of timing confusion: one day the body is told to advance, the next day it is allowed to drift back, and the result is slower progress or no clear progress at all.

People often try to fix sleep with force because the problem feels urgent. They stay in bed later to "make up" for lost sleep, then try to compensate with an early bedtime the next night. They use bright light aggressively for a few days, then stop when life gets busy. They follow a strict schedule on weekdays and abandon it on weekends. From the body's perspective, these swings are not neutral. They send mixed signals that can weaken the very adjustment you are trying to create. The clock does not need perfection, but it does need enough regularity to detect a dependable pattern.

Consistency is especially important because circadian timing changes gradually. The brain does not usually leap from one schedule to another in a single step. It shifts in response to repeated exposure, often in small increments. That means the most effective strategy is often less dramatic than people expect: a fixed wake time, a predictable morning light routine, a steady evening wind-down, and limited variation across the week. These smaller actions may look unimpressive compared with an all-out attempt to "fix" sleep in one night, but they are far more likely to produce a stable shift that lasts.

There is also a practical reason consistency works better than intensity: it is easier to sustain. Sleep changes fail most often not because the science is wrong, but because the plan is too demanding to maintain in ordinary life. A schedule that requires perfect discipline, elaborate equipment, or constant vigilance tends to collapse as soon as stress, travel, family obligations, or fatigue interfere. A simpler plan that can survive imperfect days gives the circadian system repeated chances to receive the same cue. In that sense, consistency is not about rigidity. It is about choosing a rhythm you can actually keep.

The same principle applies to light, meals, exercise, and evening behavior. A brief but regular morning walk outdoors may be more useful than a single long exposure that happens at inconsistent times. Eating breakfast at roughly the same hour each day can reinforce timing more effectively than alternating between skipped meals and heavy late-night eating. Exercise can support alertness and sleep timing, but only if its timing is reasonably steady. Even the way you handle evenings matters:

dimming lights and reducing stimulation most nights will teach the body more than a dramatic "digital detox" that happens once in a while and then disappears.

Consistency also protects against the common trap of overcorrecting. When sleep is not improving quickly, it is tempting to make the intervention stronger: earlier and earlier bedtimes, longer light sessions, more drastic schedule shifts, or repeated attempts to "catch up" on rest. But stronger is not always better. If the timing is wrong, intensity can push the system in an unhelpful direction. If the timing is right, too much force can make the routine hard to follow. The goal is not to overwhelm the clock; it is to train it.

That training effect is easiest to see when you think in terms of cues. The body does not ask whether a habit is impressive. It asks whether the cue arrives often enough to matter. A stable wake time, repeated daily, becomes a stronger signal than a perfect routine that appears only occasionally. Over time, those repeated signals shape sleep pressure, alertness, and the timing of drowsiness in a way that single efforts cannot. The more predictable the cue, the more predictable the response. And for circadian disorders, predictability is often the difference between a schedule that keeps slipping and one that begins to hold.

The importance of timing for sleep, meals, and exercise

The body clock does not respond only to light and darkness. It also listens closely to when you eat, move, and repeat those actions from one day to the next. These cues are sometimes called "time givers" because they help the body decide what part of the day it is. When they are regular, they reinforce the message already coming from light exposure and sleep timing. When they are scattered, delayed, or constantly changing, they can blur that message and make circadian adjustment harder. In other words, your schedule does not just reflect your internal clock; it helps shape it.

Meal timing is one of the clearest examples. The digestive system, liver, pancreas, and other metabolic tissues all follow daily rhythms of their own. They expect food at certain times and prepare for it by adjusting hormone release, enzyme activity, and fuel use. Eating late at night can send a confusing signal, especially if the brain is already trying to shift toward sleep mode. A heavy meal close to bedtime may also keep the body active when it should be settling down, making sleep feel lighter or more fragmented. On the other hand, a fairly consistent first meal of the day can act like a morning cue, especially when it happens soon after waking. The exact meal pattern does not need to be rigid, but it should be regular enough that the body can anticipate it.

This matters in circadian rhythm disorders because meal timing can either support the direction you want your clock to move or work against it. If you are trying to advance a delayed sleep schedule, eating very late into the evening can keep the body in a later biological pattern. If you are trying to hold an earlier schedule, skipping breakfast and pushing most calories into the late day may weaken the morning signal that helps anchor wake time. The goal is not to treat food as a cure for sleep problems, but to use it as a stabilizing cue. Regular meals help the body tell the difference between daytime activity and nighttime recovery.

Exercise works in a similar way, though the signal is a little different. Physical activity raises body temperature, increases alertness, and stimulates systems that are linked to wakefulness and energy regulation. Because of that, exercise can strengthen daytime timing when it is done consistently. Morning or daytime movement often supports a more alert daytime state and can help reinforce the idea that the day has begun. For many people, this is especially helpful when the body clock is drifting later and mornings feel foggy or unreal. Exercise becomes another reliable marker that says, in effect, this is active time.

Timing matters here as much as the exercise itself. A workout that is energizing at 8 a.m. may be too activating at 10 p.m. for someone whose sleep is already fragile. That does not mean evening exercise is always harmful. Some people tolerate it well, especially if it is moderate and ends long before bedtime. But if you notice that late workouts leave you keyed up, delay sleepiness, or make your body feel too alert at night, the timing may be part of the problem. In circadian treatment, the question is not whether exercise is good or bad in the abstract. It is whether it is happening at a time that supports the sleep schedule you are trying to build.

The most useful approach is to think in terms of consistency, not perfection. Meals and exercise do not need to occur at the exact same minute every day, but large swings can weaken their timing value. A body that eats breakfast one day, brunch the next, and nothing until late afternoon on the third day receives mixed signals about when the active phase begins. The same is true for movement. A routine that includes a predictable walk, gym session, or stretch period at roughly the same point in the day gives the circadian system another dependable cue. Over time, those repeated patterns can help the body settle into a clearer rhythm.

This is one reason behavioral change works best when it is coordinated. If you wake at a set time, seek morning light, eat at a steady hour, and move your body during the day, each action reinforces the others. The body gets a layered message: daytime has started, activity is expected, fuel is available, and sleep belongs later. That layering is especially helpful when the clock has been drifting or when you are trying to shift it in a new direction. Small routines can become biologically meaningful when they happen at the same time day after day.

It also helps to notice what undermines these cues. Grazing late at night, skipping meals and then overeating after dark, exercising sporadically at very different hours, or using food and movement only as responses to stress can all weaken timing. The issue is not moral discipline. It is signal clarity. The body clock works better when the day has a recognizable shape. Regular meals and regular movement give that shape more definition, and that makes it easier for the sleep system to know when it is supposed to be active and when it is supposed to power down.

How habits become powerful biological cues

The body learns from repetition. When the same behavior happens at the same time every day, the circadian system begins to treat it as information, not just routine. That is why habits can become powerful biological cues: over time, they stop being merely choices you make and start functioning like signals the body uses to predict what comes next. A regular wake time, a predictable first meal, a consistent walk outside, or a familiar wind-down sequence can all help the brain and body anticipate the next phase of the day. The more reliable the pattern, the more the clock can use it.

This happens because circadian timing is built to respond to patterns in the environment. The brain is not only looking for light and darkness; it is also looking for repeated daily structure. If you get up at the same hour, eat breakfast soon after, and expose yourself to morning light, those actions reinforce one another. They tell the body that daytime has begun. Later, when the same sequence in reverse appears in the evening—dimming lights, slowing activity, delaying food, and repeating a calming routine—the body receives a different message: the active part of the day is ending. In this way, ordinary habits become part of the timing system itself.

The power of habit as a biological cue depends heavily on consistency. A cue that appears once in a while is easy for the body to ignore. A cue that appears nearly every day becomes easier to trust. This is why the timing of a behavior often matters more than the behavior alone. For example, exercise can support circadian alignment, but a workout at a different hour each day sends a less stable message than movement that happens in a predictable window. Meals work the same way. Eating breakfast at roughly the same time each morning gives the body a recurring sign that the day has started, while erratic meal timing can blur the distinction between daytime and nighttime physiology.

Habits also shape the body by creating associations. If your brain learns that a certain sequence always leads to sleep, it begins to respond earlier in the sequence. Lower lighting, a warm shower, brushing your teeth, and putting away screens may not seem biologically significant on their own, but when they happen in the same order night after night, they become a learned signal for downshifting. The body starts preparing before sleep actually arrives. This is one reason people often feel sleepier once they begin a familiar bedtime routine, even if they did not feel especially tired at the start of it.

Not all habits help the clock, however. Some repeated behaviors send mixed or competing signals. Late-night snacking, bright overhead light after dark, irregular sleep-ins on weekends, or checking messages in bed can all weaken the message that night is for rest. The issue is not moral failure or lack of self-control. It is that the circadian system is receiving a confusing pattern. If one part of the day says "stay alert" and another says "prepare for sleep," the body has to guess which cue matters most. Over time, those mixed signals can make sleep timing less stable and more dependent on effort.

It is useful to think of habits as a language the body can learn. A single word does not create fluency; repeated use does. In the same way, one early bedtime or one perfect morning routine will not reset the clock by itself. What matters is the repeated message. When the same cues arrive day after day, the circadian system begins to adjust its expectations. Sleep becomes easier to predict, alertness becomes easier to organize, and the transition between day and night becomes less abrupt. The body is not being commanded into compliance; it is being trained through repetition.

This is also why small habits can have outsized effects when they are timed well. A brief walk outside soon after waking may do more for circadian alignment than a much longer walk taken late in the evening. A stable breakfast time may matter more than occasional attempts to "catch up" on sleep. Even the simple act of keeping mornings and evenings distinct can help the body sort time into categories. The goal is not perfection. It is to create enough regularity that the body can stop guessing. Once the brain has repeated evidence for when the day begins and ends, it can begin to use those habits as dependable markers of time.

Chapter 5: Using Light as a Therapeutic Tool

Light is not just something to avoid or seek out; it is one of the most precise tools available for shaping circadian timing. Because the brain reads light as a direct message about time of day, changing how and when you are exposed to it can help move sleep in the direction you need without relying on force or guesswork. That makes light management especially important when your schedule and your internal clock are out of sync. The challenge is that light works differently depending on timing, intensity, and the pattern of exposure across the day, so the same source can either support sleep or keep it from arriving when you want it.

Morning light for advancing the sleep phase

Morning light is one of the most effective tools for shifting a delayed sleep pattern earlier because it sends the brain a clear message that the day has begun. For someone whose clock runs late, the problem is often not that sleep is absent, but that the timing of sleepiness arrives too far into the night. Bright light soon after waking helps move the circadian system in the advancing direction, nudging the internal clock toward earlier sleepiness the following evening and earlier wakefulness the next morning. The effect is not immediate in the sense of making you sleepy on the spot. Instead, it works by gradually changing the timing of the signals that regulate alertness, temperature, and melatonin release.

The timing matters as much as the light itself. Morning light is most useful when it arrives soon after waking, especially in the first hour or two of the day. That early exposure tells the circadian system that the biological day has started, which helps anchor the clock earlier. If light is delayed until late morning or afternoon, the effect is less helpful for advancing the phase and may even work against the goal if it becomes part of a pattern of sleeping in and starting the day late. For people with delayed sleep phase, the temptation is often to protect the late-night sleep window by allowing a late wake time. Unfortunately, that can keep the clock set too late. A more effective strategy is to pair a consistent wake time with a reliable dose of bright light shortly afterward.

Natural outdoor light is usually the best option. Even on a cloudy day, outdoor light is far brighter than typical indoor lighting, and that brightness is what the circadian system responds to. A short walk, sitting outside with coffee or breakfast, or simply stepping into daylight after waking can be enough to begin shifting the body clock in the right direction. The key is consistency. Ten to thirty minutes of outdoor light each morning is often more useful than a longer but irregular exposure. If the weather, safety, or schedule makes outdoor light difficult, a properly used light therapy box can serve as an alternative, but the same principle applies: use it early, use it regularly, and make it part of a stable wake-up routine.

It also helps to think about what can dilute the effect of morning light. If you wake up and immediately stay in a dim room, scroll on your phone in bed, or keep curtains closed for a long stretch, the brain receives a weaker "daytime" signal. Likewise, if you wake early but remain indoors under low light for most of the morning, the circadian system may not get enough information to shift earlier. This does not mean every minute must be optimized. It does mean that the first part of the day should feel noticeably brighter than the night before. Light, movement, and a predictable first meal work well together because they all reinforce the same message: the body should be awake now.

For some people, advancing the sleep phase requires a careful balance between morning light and evening light avoidance. If you get strong light early but then expose yourself to bright light late at night, the late light can partially cancel the advance you are trying to create. That is why morning light works best when it is part of a broader timing plan. In practical terms, this means getting as much bright light as possible after waking and then reducing bright light in the hours before bed. The body clock responds to the overall pattern, not to one isolated action. A person who spends 20 minutes in strong morning light but then sits under bright LEDs until midnight is sending mixed instructions.

Some readers worry that morning light will wake them too much or make them feel uncomfortable if they are already sleep deprived. In most cases, the goal is not to create stimulation in the ordinary sense. The purpose is to realign timing, not to force alertness beyond what the body can handle. If light feels harsh, start with a manageable dose and build consistency before intensity. A brief outdoor walk may be easier than sitting still in bright light. Sunglasses should generally be avoided during the early morning exposure unless there is a medical reason to use them, because they reduce the signal reaching the brain. At the same time, safety comes first: if you are driving, walking in a dangerous area, or dealing with eye conditions that require special precautions, adjust the method rather than abandoning the approach entirely.

Advancing the sleep phase is usually a gradual process. A single morning outside will not reset a delayed clock, and that is not a failure. The circadian system changes through repeated cues, not one-time interventions. The goal is to make morning light a dependable part of the day so the brain begins to expect earlier wakefulness and earlier sleep. When that expectation takes hold, bedtime often becomes easier because the internal pressure to stay awake into the night starts to ease. Morning light does not replace good sleep habits, but it makes those habits more effective by shifting the biological timing underneath them.

Evening light reduction and screen management

Evening light has a different effect on the body clock than morning light. After sunset, the circadian system is preparing to move toward night mode, and bright light can interrupt that transition. For someone with a delayed sleep pattern, that interruption is especially important because the clock is already tending to run late. A well-lit kitchen, a bright living room, overhead LEDs, and the glow from phones, tablets, laptops, and televisions can all send the same basic message: stay alert, stay awake, keep the biological day going a little longer. The result is not just a vague sense of being "too stimulated." It is a measurable delay in the signal that helps the brain begin shifting toward sleep.

This does not mean that every light source at night is equally disruptive or that you must live in darkness. The issue is more about brightness, timing, and proximity than about light itself. A dim lamp used for a quiet activity is not the same as a bright screen held close to the face. Light that enters the eyes directly and repeatedly in the last hours before bed is the most likely to delay sleep timing. That is why evening routines should focus on lowering the overall level of illumination and reducing the most stimulating sources first. The goal is to make the environment match the message you want the body to receive: the active part of the day is ending.

Screen use deserves special attention because it combines light exposure with mental engagement. Even if the light from a device is not extremely bright, the content itself can keep the brain alert. Scrolling, gaming, answering messages, watching tense shows, or working late into the night can all prolong wakefulness for two reasons at once: the eyes are receiving a stimulating light signal, and the mind is being asked to stay involved. For that reason, screen management is not only about the device settings. It is also about deciding which activities belong close to bedtime and which do not. A relaxing audiobook or a calm, low-brightness activity may be easier on the circadian system than an endless stream of alerts, news, or social media.

One useful approach is to think in layers rather than in absolutes. Start by lowering the brightest lights in the home one to two hours before sleep, especially overhead lighting and any lights aimed directly at the face. Then reduce screen brightness and, when possible, shift to smaller, dimmer, or less immersive devices. Night mode or blue-light filters can help reduce the alerting effect of screens, but they do not erase it completely. A dimmed screen is still a screen. If your sleep is especially delayed, the safest assumption is that less screen exposure in the late evening is better than more, even when the device is set to a warmer color.

It also helps to make the bedroom a low-light zone rather than a second living room. If you need light for practical reasons, choose the least activating option available. Use a soft lamp instead of bright ceiling lights. Keep the phone out of direct view if you do not need it. Avoid checking the time repeatedly, since that often leads to more screen exposure and more mental activation than intended. If you wake during the night, try to keep the environment dark enough that the body does not interpret the moment as the start of daytime. Even brief bursts of bright light in the middle of the night can weaken the signal that sleep is supposed to continue.

For many people, the hardest part is not knowing where to draw the line. A strict rule that says "no screens after dinner" may be unrealistic in a household with work demands, family responsibilities, or a need to stay reachable. In those cases, it is better to create a realistic reduction plan than to aim for perfection and give up when that proves impossible. You might set a cutoff for the most stimulating activities, then allow a short period of low-light, low-engagement screen use if needed. You might move some tasks earlier in the evening so that the final hour before bed is calmer. You might also use environmental changes that are easier to sustain, such as dimmer bulbs, closed blinds, and a consistent wind-down location away from bright shared spaces.

The key is consistency. The body clock responds to repeated patterns, so an occasional late-night screen session is less disruptive than a nightly routine of bright light and active stimulation right before bed. If your sleep is drifting later, the evening hours are a place where small changes can have an outsized effect over time. Lowering light, reducing screen intensity, and limiting mentally activating content do not force sleep to happen. They simply stop sending the body the wrong signal at the wrong time, which makes it easier for the natural sleep drive to take over when bedtime arrives.

Choosing and using a light therapy box safely

A light therapy box can be useful when natural morning light is not available, but it should be treated as a therapeutic device, not a household lamp. The goal is to deliver a controlled dose of bright light at the right time of day so the brain receives a clear timing signal. For that reason, the most important features are brightness, spectrum, and how the light is delivered. Most clinical boxes are designed to provide about 10,000 lux at a specific distance, usually measured at the user's eye level. That does not mean you stare into the light. It means the box is bright enough, at the correct distance, to do its job while you sit nearby and go about a quiet activity such as reading, eating breakfast, or planning the day.

When choosing a box, look for one that is specifically marketed for light therapy and that filters out most ultraviolet light. UV exposure is not needed for circadian treatment and only adds risk. A larger surface area is often easier to use than a small one because it gives you more freedom to move your head slightly without losing the effect. The light should feel bright, but not harsh, and it should be stable rather than flickering. If a box has adjustable intensity, that can be helpful, especially if you are sensitive to light or are starting with shorter sessions. Some people prefer a box with a warm or neutral white appearance, but what matters most for circadian timing is brightness and consistency, not whether the light looks pleasant in the same way a room lamp does.

Placement matters as much as the box itself. The device should sit off to the side or slightly above your line of sight, not directly into your eyes. You want the light to reach your retinas while you remain comfortable enough to use it for the full session. That usually means positioning the box at the recommended distance and angling it so the light enters your eyes indirectly while you are facing the general direction of the device. Avoid closing your eyes or turning away from it, because that reduces the signal the brain receives. At the same time, do not force yourself to stare. The therapy works through exposure, not attention. Many people use the time to eat breakfast, check messages, or read, as long as the device remains within the recommended setup.

Timing is where light therapy becomes a treatment rather than a bright habit. For delayed sleep patterns, the box is usually used soon after waking, when the goal is to advance the body clock and strengthen morning alertness. For advanced sleep patterns, the timing can be different and may require more caution, because morning light can push the clock even earlier. Shift work and irregular schedules can make the situation more complex still. The same device can help one pattern and worsen another if it is used at the wrong hour. That is why light therapy should be matched to the timing problem you are trying to correct, not used simply because it feels energizing. If the timing is uncertain, it is better to get guidance than to guess.

Start conservatively if you are new to light therapy. Many people assume that more light and longer sessions will always work better, but circadian systems respond to regularity and appropriate timing more than to force. A common starting approach is a 20- to 30-minute session, though some people need more or less depending on the box, the distance, and their sensitivity. If you are using the box at the full recommended brightness, keep the session consistent from day to day rather than changing it constantly. If you notice eyestrain, headache, agitation, or an unwanted shift in sleep timing, those are signs to adjust the dose or timing. The purpose is to create a reliable signal, not to overwhelm your system.

Safety deserves as much attention as effectiveness. People with bipolar disorder, a history of mania, certain retinal conditions, or eye disease should speak with a clinician before starting light therapy. The same caution applies if you take medications that increase light sensitivity or if you have significant eye discomfort, visual changes, or migraines that seem to be triggered by brightness. If you wear glasses or contact lenses, ask whether your correction affects how the light should be positioned. It is also wise to avoid using the box when driving, operating machinery, or doing anything that requires full visual concentration. Light therapy should fit into a calm, predictable routine where you can sit still and let the exposure do its work.

It also helps to think about what light therapy is not. It is not a substitute for a stable wake time, and it does not cancel out late-night light exposure, irregular meals, or a constantly shifting schedule. A box can reinforce a new timing pattern, but it cannot fully compensate for habits that keep sending the opposite message. For that reason, the best results usually come when the session is paired with a fixed wake time, morning activity, and a clear plan for reducing evening brightness. In other words, the box is one strong cue in a larger system of cues. Used well, it can help anchor the day and make the rest of your circadian routine more effective.

Matching light timing to your specific disorder

Light therapy is most effective when it is matched to the direction you want your clock to move. That sounds simple, but it is where many people get stuck. They know light matters, yet they use it in the wrong part of the day for their specific pattern. The same bright morning light that helps a delayed sleep phase can make an advanced sleep phase worse if it is timed incorrectly. Likewise, the same evening light reduction that helps someone who falls asleep too late may be less useful for someone whose main problem is waking too early. The key is to stop thinking of light as a general sleep aid and start thinking of it as a timing signal with different effects depending on when it is delivered.

If your sleep comes too late, your goal is usually to shift the clock earlier. In that case, bright light soon after waking is the main tool. The earlier in your wake period you receive that light, the more clearly it tells the brain that day has begun. This does not mean forcing yourself outside at dawn every day if that is unrealistic, but it does mean making the first part of your morning as bright as possible. Open the blinds, step outdoors if you can, and use a light box if natural light is limited. At the same time, reduce strong light late in the evening, especially in the two to three hours before bed. The combination matters: morning light pushes the clock earlier, while evening darkness helps prevent it from drifting later again.

For delayed sleep phase, consistency is more important than perfection. A single bright morning will not reset the clock if the rest of the week is filled with late-night light exposure and sleeping in. Try to keep the wake time steady, because the timing of morning light depends on when you actually wake up. If your schedule varies by several hours, the light signal becomes less precise. You do not need to create a harsh, artificial environment all day; instead, focus on making the morning brighter and the evening dimmer. Many people benefit from adding a brief outdoor walk within the first hour after waking, then using lower indoor light levels and reduced screen brightness after sunset. The goal is to make the day feel clearly like day and the night feel clearly like night.

If your sleep comes too early, the logic changes. Advanced sleep phase is often helped by delaying the clock rather than advancing it. In practical terms, that means evening light can be useful, especially later in the day, because it helps hold the clock back and reduce the pull toward early sleepiness. Bright light in the late afternoon or evening may help extend alertness into the desired bedtime window. Morning light, by contrast, may reinforce an already early clock and make early waking even more likely. That does not mean you should avoid all daylight after sunrise, but it does mean you may need to be more cautious about very bright early-morning exposure if your sleep is already arriving too soon.

People with advanced sleep phase often make the mistake of trying to “fix” early waking by going to bed even earlier, which usually shortens the day without solving the timing problem. A better approach is to protect the evening from becoming too quiet and too dark too soon. Keep the lights reasonably bright in the hours before bedtime, stay engaged in alerting activities, and avoid drifting to bed at the first sign of evening sleepiness unless that is truly your target bedtime. If you use light strategically, the aim is not to force yourself into artificial wakefulness all night. It is to prevent the circadian system from ending the day too soon.

Shift work and rotating schedules require a different kind of judgment because the "right" light timing depends on the schedule you are trying to support. If you are working overnight and need to stay alert during the night shift, bright light during the shift can improve alertness and help the body adapt to the temporary schedule. But that same light may make it harder to sleep after work if you keep exposing yourself to strong daylight on the way home. In that case, the problem is not light itself but the sequence of light exposures. You may need bright light at work, then sunglasses or reduced light on the commute, followed by a dark sleep environment during the daytime sleep period. The goal is to separate the work period from the sleep period as clearly as possible.

For jet lag, the correct light timing depends on whether you are traveling east or west and how many time zones you crossed. Eastward travel usually requires the clock to move earlier, so morning light at the destination becomes especially helpful, while late-evening light may slow adjustment. Westward travel usually requires a delay, so later-day light can help extend wakefulness and reduce the feeling that bedtime is arriving too soon. Because travel schedules are often messy, the most practical strategy is to anchor light to the local clock as soon as possible after arrival. Even a few well-timed outdoor sessions can help the brain begin treating the destination as the new day.

In every case, the principle is the same: match light to the direction of change you need. Morning light tends to advance the clock, evening light tends to delay it, and the wrong timing can work against you even if the light is otherwise healthy. That is why it helps to think in terms of your specific disorder rather than in terms of generic sleep advice. If you are trying to fall asleep earlier, brighten the beginning of your day and dim the end of it. If you are trying to stay awake later, strengthen light later in the day and avoid making mornings too intense. If your schedule is imposed by work or travel, use light to support the sleep period you actually need, not the one your body would choose on its own. The more precisely you match timing to pattern, the less effort it takes to get a meaningful response.

Chapter 6: Building a Sleep Schedule That Actually Works

Once light exposure is working in your favor, the next step is to make your daily sleep schedule easier for the body to follow. Circadian change tends to hold when the day is organized around a few dependable anchors, because the brain responds best to repeated patterns rather than occasional bursts of effort. This is where schedule design matters: not as a rigid form of discipline, but as a way of reducing mixed signals that keep sleep timing unstable. A workable schedule gives your body a clearer expectation of when the day begins, when winding down starts, and how much variation it should tolerate from one night to the next.

Setting a fixed wake time as the anchor

A fixed wake time is the most reliable anchor in a circadian schedule because it gives the body one daily event it can count on, no matter how the previous night went. Sleep timing is influenced by many variables, but wake time is the point where the day is forced to begin. When that point stays consistent, it becomes easier for the brain to organize the rest of the 24-hour cycle around it. If wake time shifts from day to day, the body receives mixed information: sometimes morning starts at 6:30, sometimes at 9:00, sometimes after a long lie-in. That variability makes it harder for the internal clock to predict when sleep should arrive later that night.

This is especially important for people whose sleep is delayed. A late bedtime often leads to a late wake time, and a late wake time tends to preserve the delay. Even if you fall asleep at 2:00 a.m., sleeping until late morning can keep your circadian system set to a later schedule. The same pattern can happen in reverse for people with advanced sleep phase: going to bed early and waking very early may reinforce an early clock that keeps shifting the whole rhythm forward. In both cases, the wake time is not just the end of sleep. It is a signal that helps define the next cycle.

That does not mean you should force yourself out of bed after a severely short night and expect everything to improve immediately. The purpose of a fixed wake time is not punishment, and it is not a test of toughness. It is a timing cue. If you had a poor night, you may feel tired the next day, but keeping the wake time steady still helps prevent the clock from drifting further. Over time, that consistency can reduce the gap between when you want to sleep and when you actually become sleepy. The body often responds better to a stable schedule repeated across many days than to occasional attempts to “catch up” with a long sleep-in.

To make a fixed wake time work, choose a time you can realistically maintain on both workdays and days off. The best anchor is not the ideal time on paper; it is the time you can actually keep most days of the week. If your schedule demands a 7:00 a.m. rise on weekdays, then that time should usually remain your wake time on weekends as well. If you choose a wake time that is too ambitious, you are more likely to fail at it and then swing late on the next day off, which weakens the signal. Consistency matters more than perfection, and a stable average matters more than a flawless but short-lived effort.

It also helps to treat wake time as the first active step in the day rather than the moment you feel fully alert. For many people with circadian misalignment, alertness arrives gradually after waking. The body may need light exposure, movement, food, and a little time before it feels fully online. That is normal. The goal is not to wait until you feel ready to get up; the goal is to use getting up at the same time as the cue that starts the rest of the day. Once you are awake, the body can begin receiving the daytime signals that reinforce the schedule.

A fixed wake time becomes even more powerful when it is paired with a predictable first hour. Try to make the first part of the morning look similar from day to day: get out of bed, open the blinds or go outside, keep light exposure regular, and avoid drifting back into bed or lying in darkness for long periods. If you use an alarm, place it far enough away that you must stand up to turn it off. If you tend to snooze repeatedly, reduce the opportunity for a fragmented morning, because repeated dozing can blur the message that the day has begun. The more clearly the body receives that message, the easier it is for the rest of the schedule to settle.

There will be days when life interferes. Travel, illness, late obligations, or family demands can all disrupt the anchor. When that happens, return to the fixed wake time as soon as you reasonably can instead of letting one late morning turn into several. A single deviation is less damaging than a pattern of drift. The broader goal is to make your wake time the most dependable part of the day, because that one stable point gives every other habit a place to attach. Bedtime, meals, light exposure, exercise, and evening wind-down all become easier to regulate when the body knows, with repeated certainty, when morning begins.

Creating a bedtime routine that signals sleep

A bedtime routine works best when it does more than fill time before bed. It should act as a repeated signal that tells the brain the active part of the day is ending and the sleep period is approaching. For people with circadian rhythm problems, this signal matters because the body often needs help distinguishing "late evening" from "still time to stay alert." A routine that is calm, predictable, and repeated in the same order each night can become one of the clearest cues that sleep is near.

The most effective routines are not necessarily the longest or most elaborate ones. In fact, a routine that is too complicated can become another source of stress, especially if you miss a step and feel as though you have failed at sleep. The goal is not perfection. The goal is repetition. When the same sequence happens night after night, the brain begins to connect those steps with reduced activity, lower stimulation, and a shift toward rest. Over time, the routine itself becomes part of the timing system.

To work as a sleep signal, the routine should begin before you are already exhausted. If you wait until you are overwhelmed by sleepiness, you are more likely to rush through the process or skip it entirely. Instead, think of the routine as a bridge between daytime and sleep. That bridge can be short. For some people, it may be 20 minutes; for others, 45 minutes or more. What matters is that it happens at roughly the same time each night and leads the body through the same general sequence of events.

Start by reducing stimulation in a deliberate way. Bright overhead light, loud conversation, work email, emotionally charged content, and demanding tasks all keep the nervous system in a more alert state. A bedtime routine should gradually move away from those signals. Dim the lights, lower the volume of your environment, and choose activities that do not require intense focus. If screens are part of your evening, use them with intention rather than as a default source of stimulation. The point is not that every screen must disappear instantly, but that the brain should receive a consistent message that the day is winding down.

Many people benefit from a routine built around a few familiar actions: washing up, changing into sleep clothes, preparing for the next day, and spending a few quiet minutes doing something repetitive and low effort. Reading a paper book, gentle stretching, light journaling, or a brief breathing exercise can all fit into this window if they feel calming rather than activating. The specific activities matter less than the fact that they are easy to repeat and not emotionally charged. If an activity makes you more engaged, more curious, or more likely to stay up longer, it is probably not serving as a sleep cue.

It also helps to make the routine distinct from the rest of the evening. If you do the same things you do during the day—sorting tasks, planning tomorrow in detail, checking messages, or moving from one stimulating activity to another—the brain does not get a clear boundary. A sleep routine should feel like a transition, not a continuation. Even small changes can help create that boundary: turning down lights in a specific order, using the same scent or tea if it is noncaffeinated, or listening to the same quiet audio each night. Repeated cues are powerful because they are easy for the body to recognize.

Consistency matters most when your schedule is unstable or your sleep has been drifting late. On those nights, it can be tempting to "make up for it" by staying up later and then trying to crash into sleep all at once. That usually works against circadian adjustment. A better approach is to keep the wind-down sequence anchored to the bedtime you are trying to establish, even if sleep does not arrive immediately. The routine is not a guarantee of instant sleep; it is a signal that supports the timing system over time. If you train the body to expect the same pattern, sleep becomes easier to approach at the right hour.

It can be useful to think of your bedtime routine as a set of instructions for the nervous system: lower the light, lower the pace, lower the demands. The more often those instructions are repeated in the same order, the more the body learns to respond before you are consciously sleepy. That learned response is especially valuable in circadian disorders, where the challenge is often not simply falling asleep, but teaching sleep to arrive at a more workable time. A steady routine gives the brain one more reliable marker that night has begun.

Avoiding the trap of weekend sleep swings

Weekend sleep swings are one of the most common ways people accidentally undo the work they do during the week. After several days of early alarms, limited sleep, or strict routines, it is tempting to treat Saturday and Sunday as a chance to "catch up" by sleeping late, staying up later, or doing both. The problem is that the body clock does not experience the weekend as a reward system. It experiences it as a change in time cues. A two-hour sleep-in may feel harmless, but if it happens every week, the brain begins to receive a different message about when morning starts, when daytime begins, and when night is supposed to end.

That shift can be especially disruptive for people trying to move a delayed sleep pattern earlier. Sleeping late on free days often pushes the circadian system later, making Sunday night harder and Monday morning more difficult. Even if the extra sleep feels restorative in the moment, it can create a recurring cycle: short or structured sleep during the week, then a late wake time on the weekend, then a later bedtime, then another Monday struggle. The result is not true recovery so much as a weekly mini-jet lag. Each Monday becomes a reset that never quite resets in the right direction.

The same issue can affect people with advanced sleep phase, but in a different way. If sleepiness arrives early and waking happens before dawn, a person may use the weekend to stay up much later in an effort to reclaim evening hours. That can seem reasonable, but it often produces a similar mismatch. The body clock has already shifted early, so extending the evening dramatically may leave the person overtired, fragmented, or groggy the next day. In either case, the problem is not simply the amount of sleep. It is the irregular timing of sleep and wake signals, which weakens the stability the circadian system depends on.

A better approach is to protect the anchor points that matter most. Wake time is usually the strongest anchor, so the goal is to keep it as close as possible to the weekday schedule, even on days off. If you need more sleep, it is usually better to allow a modest extension rather than a large swing. For example, if your weekday wake time is 6:30 a.m., sleeping until 7:30 or 8:00 a.m. may be manageable, while sleeping until 10:30 or 11:00 a.m. is much more likely to push your clock later. The same principle applies to bedtime: a small shift may be tolerable, but a dramatic weekend delay can erase the progress you made during the week.

It also helps to think about how weekend behaviors reinforce the message of "day" and "night." Late-night light, casual snacking, alcohol, and long naps can all make it easier to drift away from a stable rhythm. If you stay up later on Friday and Saturday, then sleep in and nap on Saturday and Sunday, the body gets a confusing set of cues that can weaken the pressure to sleep at the right time on Sunday night. You do not need a perfect weekend to protect your rhythm, but you do need enough consistency that the body can still tell what time it is.

If social plans are the reason your schedule shifts, it may help to choose one or two routines that stay fixed no matter what. Some people preserve the same wake time and morning light exposure, then allow a slightly later bedtime only once or twice a week. Others keep the same breakfast timing and outdoor walk, even if the rest of the day changes. These smaller anchors can reduce the amount of circadian drift caused by weekend variability. The goal is not to eliminate flexibility. It is to keep flexibility from turning into a pattern that repeatedly pushes the clock in the wrong direction.

There is also an important mindset shift here. Weekend sleep swings often happen because people are trying to make up for sleep debt, but the body usually responds better to steadiness than to dramatic compensation. If you are consistently exhausted by Friday, that is a sign to look at the weekday schedule itself rather than relying on the weekend to repair it. A more stable sleep window, a slightly earlier bedtime, or a more realistic wake time may do more for your long-term energy than any amount of sleeping in. The best weekend is not the one that feels most different from the workweek. It is the one that gives you enough rest without teaching your body clock to start over every Monday.

Adjusting schedules gradually instead of abruptly

When you need to shift sleep timing, the safest approach is usually to move it in small steps rather than by force. The circadian system does not respond well to sudden demands, especially if the change asks the body to fall asleep much earlier or much later than it has been doing. A dramatic shift may look efficient on paper, but in practice it often creates a worse mismatch: you lie in bed awake, wake up unrefreshed, and end up reinforcing the very pattern you were trying to change. Gradual adjustment gives the brain time to accept the new schedule as normal instead of treating it as an emergency.

This matters because sleep is not controlled by a single switch. It is the result of several timing signals lining up at once: light exposure, wake time, meals, activity, and the pressure that builds the longer you stay awake. If you try to move bedtime by two or three hours all at once, those signals may not move together. Your alarm may say one thing, your appetite may say another, and your brain may still be following the old timing pattern. A slower shift reduces that conflict. The body can start to learn the new timing before the change becomes large enough to feel disruptive.

In most cases, the easiest place to begin is with wake time, not bedtime. If your goal is to sleep earlier, moving wake time earlier in small increments often helps the rest of the schedule follow. If your goal is to sleep later, a slightly later wake time may be part of the adjustment, but only if it does not create chaos in the rest of your day. A shift of 15 to 30 minutes every few days is often easier to tolerate than a sudden jump. The exact pace matters less than the consistency. Each step should be large enough to matter, but small enough that you can actually hold it.

It helps to think of the process as teaching the body a new pattern rather than correcting it overnight. For example, someone who is falling asleep at 1:30 a.m. and needs to be asleep closer to 11:30 p.m. may do better by moving bedtime and wake time earlier in stages. That might mean going to bed 15 minutes earlier for several nights, then another 15 minutes earlier once the first change feels stable. The same idea applies in the opposite direction for advanced sleep phase, where the goal is to keep evening sleepiness from arriving too soon. Small, repeated changes are easier for the circadian system to encode than a one-time overhaul.

During these shifts, consistency is more important than perfection. If you move your schedule earlier on weekdays but let it slide back on weekends, the body receives mixed information and the adjustment slows down. The same is true if you change the clock times but keep everything else the same. A new bedtime without a new light pattern, or a new wake time without a corresponding change in morning behavior, may not be enough to move the rhythm. The schedule works best when the surrounding cues move with it: light, meals, activity, and wind-down habits should all support the same direction of change.

There is also a psychological advantage to gradual change. Abrupt schedule shifts often feel like deprivation, which makes them hard to maintain. Small changes feel more manageable, and manageable changes are more likely to become stable habits. That matters because circadian improvement depends on repetition. A schedule that you can follow for several weeks is more useful than a more aggressive plan that collapses after three days. The aim is not to prove discipline. It is to create a timing pattern the body can actually adopt.

When adjusting gradually, track the response instead of assuming every step is working equally well. Some people find that a 15-minute shift is enough to start moving sleep in the desired direction, while others need a slower pace. Watch for signs that the change is too fast: prolonged sleep-onset trouble, worsening morning grogginess, irritability, or a feeling that you are constantly fighting the clock. Those signs do not necessarily mean the schedule is wrong. They may simply mean the body needs more time at each step before moving again. A slower pace is not a failure; it is often the difference between a temporary effort and a lasting reset.

Chapter 7: Daily Habits That Strengthen Circadian Rhythm

Once your sleep schedule is anchored, the next layer of circadian support comes from the ordinary choices that fill the rest of the day. The body clock is not shaped only by light and bedtime; it also takes cues from when you eat, move, pause, and re-engage with the world around you. Those cues can either reinforce the timing you are trying to build or quietly pull it off course. This is why daily habits matter so much: they turn a good schedule into a livable one and help the brain recognize a pattern it can trust.

Meal timing and its effect on body clocks

What you eat matters, but when you eat can matter just as much. The body does not process food on a neutral clock. Digestive activity, insulin response, temperature regulation, and the release of metabolic hormones all follow daily rhythms, which means meals act as timing cues for the circadian system. A regular eating pattern helps reinforce the difference between active daytime biology and nighttime rest biology. Irregular eating does the opposite: it can blur that distinction and make it harder for the body to know when to expect energy, when to store fuel, and when to begin shifting toward sleep.

This is one reason late-night eating can be so disruptive. A large meal close to bedtime asks the body to do several things at once that are not well aligned with sleep: digest food, regulate blood sugar, and manage the rise in body temperature that often follows eating. For someone trying to fall asleep, that can create a state of internal activity at exactly the wrong time. Even if the meal does not fully wake you, it can delay the transition into nighttime physiology. People often notice this as feeling physically heavy, too warm, or strangely alert after eating late, followed by lighter sleep or a harder time falling asleep.

Meal timing can also push the clock in the other direction. A very delayed first meal, repeated day after day, may make the body treat morning as a continuation of the night. If breakfast is skipped until late morning or early afternoon, the usual daytime signals that help establish alertness may arrive too late to support a stable rhythm. For people with delayed sleep phase tendencies, this can be especially important because the whole pattern already leans late. A consistent first meal soon after waking gives the body another daytime cue that says, in effect, the active period has begun. It does not replace light, but it can strengthen the message.

Regularity matters as much as clock time. The circadian system responds best when meals happen at roughly the same points in the day, not when eating becomes a moving target. A body that receives food at predictable times can begin to anticipate digestion and metabolism more efficiently. That predictability helps peripheral clocks in the liver, gut, and other tissues stay better aligned with the master clock in the brain. When meal timing drifts from one day to the next, those peripheral clocks may become less synchronized, which can contribute to grogginess, energy swings, and a general sense that the body is never quite on schedule.

For shift workers and people with irregular schedules, meal timing can become one of the clearest ways to reduce confusion in the system. If sleep timing has to change, keeping meals anchored as much as possible can provide at least one stable reference point. The reverse is also true: eating at highly variable hours can make an already unstable schedule harder to manage. A person who works nights, snacks throughout the shift, and then eats a large meal right before trying to sleep may be sending mixed signals to the body about whether it is day or night. Even if sleep cannot be perfectly normalized, more deliberate meal timing can reduce some of that biological conflict.

It also helps to distinguish between eating enough and eating at the right time. Skipping meals in an effort to "reset" the clock is not usually helpful, and for some people it backfires by increasing stress, overeating later, or making sleep more fragmented. The goal is not to impose strict rules that make daily life harder. It is to create a pattern that supports the timing you want. For many people, that means a steady daytime eating window, a first meal that is not excessively delayed, and a final meal that leaves enough distance before bed for digestion to quiet down.

Alcohol and heavy late snacks deserve special attention because they can interfere with both sleep quality and circadian timing. Alcohol may make a person feel sleepy at first, but it often fragments sleep later in the night and can shift the body away from a clean transition into rest. Heavy, high-fat, or highly stimulating foods late in the evening can also keep the digestive system active longer than is ideal. If you are trying to move your clock earlier, the simplest habit is often to make dinner earlier and keep the last food intake modest enough that bedtime is not competing with digestion.

The practical question is not whether every meal must be perfect. It is whether your eating pattern is reinforcing the same time cues your sleep plan is trying to build. When meals occur at consistent times, during the part of the day you want to strengthen, they become useful signals. When they are scattered, delayed, or concentrated late at night, they can pull the body in the opposite direction. In circadian treatment, food is not just fuel. It is part of the timing language the body uses to decide what time it is.

Exercise timing for alertness and recovery

Exercise is one of the most useful circadian tools you can use because it influences both alertness and sleep pressure. A well-timed workout can help you feel more awake when you need to function and more ready to recover when the day is done. But exercise is not neutral in its timing. The same activity can either support your sleep schedule or make it harder to settle, depending on when it happens, how intense it is, and how sensitive your system is to stimulation. For that reason, the goal is not simply to move more. It is to place movement at the hour when it best serves the clock you are trying to build.

In general, daytime exercise tends to strengthen wakefulness. Movement raises body temperature, increases circulation, and activates the nervous system in ways that can improve focus and energy. For many people with delayed sleep timing, exercise earlier in the day can be especially helpful because it reinforces the idea that the active part of the day begins in the morning, not late in the afternoon or evening. A brisk walk, a steady bike ride, strength training, or a more structured workout can all serve this purpose. The exact form matters less than the consistency of the timing. When exercise becomes part of the same daily window, it starts to function as another cue that helps organize the day.

Morning and early afternoon exercise are usually the safest choices when your goal is to feel more alert without interfering with sleep. If you are trying to shift your rhythm earlier, physical activity soon after waking can work alongside morning light to reinforce the new timing. It can also help counter the grogginess that often appears when your body clock is still lagging behind your desired schedule. Even a moderate session can be enough to improve daytime alertness, especially if it is repeated at roughly the same time each day. The benefit is not only physical. Exercise also creates a psychological boundary between sleep and wakefulness, which can be valuable when your schedule has felt blurred or unstable.

That said, exercise is not always a problem at night. Many people can work out in the evening without any trouble, especially if the session is moderate and ends well before bedtime. Others find that even a late workout leaves them too energized to fall asleep easily. The difference often comes down to intensity, timing, and individual sensitivity. A hard interval session, heavy lifting close to bedtime, or a competitive sport that leaves you mentally keyed up may delay the transition into sleep. By contrast, lighter movement such as stretching, easy walking, or gentle yoga may help the body unwind. If you notice that evening exercise leaves you restless, hot, or mentally alert for longer than you want, treat that as useful information rather than a personal failure.

Recovery matters just as much as stimulation. Exercise is only helpful when the body has enough time to repair tissue, restore energy stores, and settle the nervous system afterward. That is one reason timing should be matched to your sleep needs rather than used to chase exhaustion. Many people assume that harder exercise will automatically improve sleep because it makes them tired. Sometimes it does, but fatigue is not the same as healthy sleep drive. If a workout is too late, too intense, or too frequent without recovery, it can leave you physically worn out while still biologically activated. The result is a body that feels depleted but not ready for sleep. Good recovery protects the circadian benefits of exercise by making sure movement supports the rhythm instead of overwhelming it.

If your schedule is irregular, try to protect one or two reliable movement anchors rather than aiming for a perfect fitness plan. A short morning walk, a lunch break stretch session, or a consistent after-work workout can all help the body recognize repeating patterns. The point is not to build an ideal athlete's routine. It is to give the circadian system something stable to expect. Regularity is especially valuable for shift workers and people with delayed sleep phase because it can prevent the day from becoming a series of random energy spikes. Even when sleep is imperfect, a predictable exercise window can help preserve a clearer distinction between active time and rest time.

It also helps to think about exercise as part of the larger timing picture. If you are using morning light to shift earlier, pairing it with movement can strengthen the signal. If you are trying to avoid evening stimulation, a late workout may work against the quieting effect you need before bed. If you are recovering from a poor night of sleep, a lighter session may be more useful than forcing a strenuous one, especially if the goal is to stay functional without pushing your system into overload. In other words, exercise should be chosen not only for fitness goals but also for timing goals. The best exercise plan for circadian health is the one that leaves you more alert when you need alertness and more recoverable when you need sleep.

Caffeine, alcohol, and other timing disruptors

Caffeine is one of the most common ways people accidentally keep their body clock from settling into a stable rhythm. Its main effect is not to create energy, but to block adenosine, a chemical that builds the pressure to sleep across the day. When that pressure is reduced too late, the result is often familiar: you may feel functional in the evening, but the cost shows up later when sleep becomes lighter, delayed, or more fragmented. For someone already dealing with delayed timing, caffeine can make the problem look like simple insomnia when it is really a timing issue being reinforced by stimulation.

The timing of caffeine matters more than many people realize. A morning cup may be harmless or even helpful for alertness, but caffeine taken in the afternoon or evening can still be active at bedtime. Its effects vary from person to person, and some people metabolize it slowly enough that even a midafternoon dose can linger into the night. That is why the question is not just how much caffeine you use, but when your last dose occurs relative to your target sleep window. If you are trying to move sleep earlier, caffeine late in the day can quietly work against that effort by making the brain feel less ready for rest at the exact time you want to build sleepiness.

It is also worth noticing the hidden sources. Coffee is obvious, but tea, cola, energy drinks, pre-workout supplements, chocolate, and some pain relievers all contain caffeine. In a circadian plan, these smaller sources can matter because they are easy to overlook and tend to be consumed at the very times when people are trying to push through fatigue. That pattern can become self-reinforcing: the later you stay up, the more you reach for caffeine, and the more caffeine you use, the later sleep tends to drift. Breaking that loop often requires choosing a cutoff time and making it consistent enough for your body to learn.

Alcohol creates a different kind of timing problem. Many people think of it as a sleep aid because it can make them feel drowsy at first, but the sleep it produces is usually less stable than natural sleep. Alcohol can shorten the time it takes to fall asleep while also increasing awakenings later in the night, reducing sleep quality, and interfering with the normal progression through sleep stages. It can also worsen snoring and breathing disruption in people who are already vulnerable to sleep apnea or upper-airway collapse. So even when alcohol seems to help you get to sleep, it may still be degrading the part of the night that matters most for restoration.

Alcohol is especially disruptive when it is used close to bedtime. The body has to process it during the same period when it is trying to move into nighttime biology, and that creates mixed signals. The result can be a night that feels sedating at the start but unsteady afterward, with more awakenings, more dehydration, and a greater chance of waking too early. For people with advanced sleep phase, alcohol may deepen the tendency to fall asleep early but still leave sleep less refreshing. For people with delayed sleep phase, it may seem to help with late-night relaxation while actually making the sleep window more fragile and less predictable.

Other timing disruptors are less obvious but work in the same direction: nicotine, late heavy meals, intense late-evening exercise, and stimulant medications taken at the wrong hour can all shift alertness when the body is trying to power down. Nicotine is a stimulant and can delay sleep onset, especially if used in the evening. Large or very late meals can keep the digestive system active when the body should be preparing for rest. Even if the food itself is healthy, the timing may be enough to push sleep later or make sleep less comfortable. The general principle is simple: anything that increases arousal, digestion, or metabolic activity late in the day can interfere with the transition into nighttime mode.

Some of these disruptors are especially important because they are socially normalized. A drink after dinner, a cup of tea to unwind, a late dessert, or a "just one more" coffee during a long workday can seem minor in isolation. But circadian timing is shaped by repetition, not intention. If these habits happen often enough, the body begins to expect stimulation at the same hour it should be learning to slow down. That is why changing timing usually works better than trying to rely on willpower at bedtime. The goal is not to make every evening rigid, but to reduce the signals that tell the brain to stay alert when you want it to move toward sleep.

When you are trying to reset your clock, it helps to think in terms of protected hours. The later the evening gets, the more important it becomes to avoid substances and behaviors that keep the system activated. A practical starting point is to identify the latest time you can use caffeine without affecting sleep, then move that cutoff earlier if needed. The same logic applies to alcohol and other stimulants: if sleep is the priority, keep the hours before bed as quiet and predictable as possible. The body responds best when the message is clear, and one of the clearest messages you can send is that the end of the day is truly ending.

Naps, stress, and social habits that affect sleep

Naps can be helpful, but they can also quietly work against the sleep pattern you are trying to build. The main issue is not that a nap is "bad" in itself. It is that daytime sleep reduces the pressure to sleep later, and that pressure is one of the forces that helps you fall asleep at the right time. If you already struggle with delayed sleep, a long or late nap can make bedtime even harder by taking the edge off sleepiness before night arrives. If you tend to fall asleep too early, an unplanned nap may deepen the feeling of evening fatigue and make the day feel even shorter. In both cases, the question is not simply whether you napped, but when, how long, and how often.

Short naps are usually less disruptive than long ones, especially if they happen early in the day. A brief nap can improve alertness, reduce sleep debt, and help you function without forcing you into a recovery cycle that lasts all afternoon. But once naps become long enough to enter deeper sleep, waking up can be groggier and the nap can leave a stronger imprint on the rest of the day. For people with circadian rhythm disorders, that matters because the goal is not just to feel less tired in the moment. The goal is to keep the internal clock receiving a clear message about when sleep belongs. A nap that blurs that message can make the next night more difficult, even if it feels necessary at the time.

Stress affects sleep in a different but equally important way. When the nervous system is under strain, the body often behaves as if it needs to stay on alert, even when the clock says it is time to rest. That state can show up as a racing mind, physical tension, shallow breathing, or a sense that you are exhausted but unable to settle. Stress does not just make bedtime unpleasant; it can also shift your timing. People under chronic stress often drift later because the evening becomes the first quiet space in the day, or because they seek relief through scrolling, snacking, or staying up "just a little longer" for personal time. Others become so drained that they fall asleep earlier than intended, then wake too early with a sense of alarm already built into the system.

That is why stress management is part of circadian care, not a separate wellness topic. The body needs a reliable transition from daytime activation to nighttime downshifting. If your evenings are filled with unresolved work, difficult conversations, or constant digital stimulation, the nervous system may never get the signal that it is safe to power down. Even when the bedroom is dark and the schedule is fixed, a stressed body can remain biologically prepared for vigilance. In practical terms, this means that sleep improvement often depends on reducing the number of hours spent in a heightened state, not just on improving the final hour before bed. A calmer evening is not a luxury; it is part of the timing system.

Social habits can either support or undermine that transition. Late dinners, long conversations, unpredictable outings, and repeated "one more episode" evenings all send the message that nighttime is still active time. The problem is not social connection itself. Human beings are social by nature, and relationships matter for mental health. The issue is timing. If your social life regularly pushes bedtime later, your body will begin to treat late hours as normal waking hours. That can be especially difficult for someone trying to advance sleep timing, because the clock is already being asked to move earlier while social habits keep pulling it back. Even pleasant activities can become circadian disruptors when they consistently delay the end of the day.

Alcohol deserves special caution here because it often appears social and relaxing while still interfering with sleep quality and timing. A drink may make the evening feel smoother, but it does not create restorative sleep. It can fragment sleep later in the night, worsen early waking, and reduce the quality of the transition into deeper rest. Caffeine used late in the day can create a similar mismatch by keeping the brain alert long after the body is ready to slow down. Nicotine, stimulating social media use, and emotionally charged late-night interactions can also keep the system activated. These habits do not merely delay bedtime; they can condition the brain to expect stimulation at the very hour it should be learning to disengage.

The most useful question to ask is whether a habit is helping your body recognize night or confusing it about what time it is. A nap taken before midafternoon, a brief stress-reduction break, or an early evening social plan may fit well within a stable circadian routine. But repeated late naps, unresolved stress carried into bed, and social patterns that extend wakefulness deep into the night all send mixed signals. If your sleep timing is already fragile, those mixed signals matter more than they would for someone with a more flexible rhythm. Protecting sleep is not only about what happens in the bedroom. It is also about how you manage the hours that lead up to it.

That often means making a few deliberate choices: keep naps brief and earlier when possible, use stress-reduction habits before the evening becomes urgent, and set social boundaries that preserve your sleep window instead of constantly shrinking it. A consistent rhythm does not require isolation or perfect self-control. It requires enough predictability that your brain can learn when the active part of the day ends. When naps, stress, and social habits are aligned with that goal, they stop competing with sleep and start supporting it.

Chapter 8: When Sleep Won't Cooperate: Problem-Solving Common Obstacles

When sleep keeps slipping away from the plan, the problem is often not a lack of effort but a mismatch between the schedule you want and the conditions your body is actually living through. Circadian change is easier when days are predictable, but real life rarely stays that neat. Travel, changing obligations, overnight work, family demands, and the occasional bad night can all interrupt even a well-built routine. That does not mean the clock is ruined or that progress has been lost. It means the plan has to be flexible enough to survive disruption without abandoning the timing cues that were helping.

What to do when your schedule keeps changing

When your schedule keeps changing, the first problem is not sleep itself but the loss of predictability. The body clock works best when it can learn what happens next. If wake time, meals, light exposure, and bedtime all shift from one day to the next, the brain gets mixed messages and has a harder time settling into a stable rhythm. In that situation, the goal is not to create a perfect schedule. It is to preserve a few dependable signals even when the rest of the day is unstable.

The most useful move is to protect one anchor that stays as consistent as possible. For many people, that anchor is the wake time, because once the day begins, it becomes easier to shape light exposure, meals, movement, and evening wind-down around it. If your work, family duties, or social obligations force different bedtimes, a steady wake time still gives the circadian system a repeated reference point. If wake time cannot be fixed every day, then choose the next most reliable cue and keep it as steady as you can. The body does not need every cue to be perfect, but it does need some cues to remain recognizable.

It also helps to think in terms of minimum standards rather than ideal routines. On a stable day, you may be able to get morning light, eat breakfast at a regular hour, exercise, and follow a full bedtime routine. On a disrupted day, you may only be able to preserve one or two of those signals. That still matters. A brief outdoor light exposure after waking, a consistent first meal, or a short wind-down sequence before sleep can all help the body understand that the day is following a familiar pattern, even if the details are not ideal. Small repetitions are more valuable than occasional perfect days followed by complete inconsistency.

When the schedule changes, avoid treating every disruption as a reason to abandon the plan. People often respond to one late night or one early meeting by shifting the entire next day, then the day after that, and soon the rhythm becomes even more unstable. If you slept later than usual, do not automatically push bedtime later just because you feel less sleepy in the evening. If you had to wake earlier than usual, do not assume you must "make up" the lost sleep by sleeping far into the next morning. Large corrections often create a second disruption that is harder to recover from than the first. The body usually does better with a return to the usual anchor as soon as possible.

Light becomes especially important when your schedule is moving around. If your day starts earlier than usual, getting some bright light soon after waking can help the body register that the active part of the day has begun, even if the timing feels off. If your evening is running late, reducing bright indoor light and screen exposure can help prevent the clock from being pushed later than it already is. In an unstable schedule, light is not just a treatment tool; it is a way of drawing a boundary between day and night when the calendar no longer does that for you.

Meals and activity can serve the same purpose. A consistent first meal, even if it is small, tells the body that daytime metabolism has started. Regular movement, even if it is only a short walk, reinforces the sense that the day is underway. These cues are especially useful when work hours, travel, caregiving, or rotating commitments prevent a normal sleep pattern. The more your schedule changes, the more important it becomes to repeat the signals that are still under your control. You may not be able to control the timing of every obligation, but you can often control the order in which you expose yourself to light, food, movement, and rest.

It is also wise to decide in advance which disruptions deserve flexibility and which ones should not change the rest of your week. A single late event does not always require a new sleep schedule. A one-night emergency, an unexpected meeting, or a family obligation may be unavoidable, but the recovery plan should be simple: return to your usual wake time, get light early, avoid drifting too late the next night, and resume your normal cues the following day. The less you improvise in the moment, the less likely you are to turn a temporary change into a lasting pattern.

When your schedule keeps changing often, the aim is not to force the body clock into perfect alignment every day. It is to reduce the amount of confusion the clock has to absorb. Protect the anchors you can protect. Repeat the cues you can repeat. Keep the changes small when you have a choice, and recover quickly when you do not. A schedule that changes frequently will always make circadian stability harder, but it does not make it impossible. The more consistently you preserve a few reliable signals, the more the body has to work with, even in an unpredictable life.

Managing sleep shifts during travel and time zone changes

Travel disrupts sleep because it changes several timing cues at once. The clock on the wall moves, but so do light exposure, meal times, activity patterns, and the pressure to sleep. A flight that seems short in real time can still leave the body dealing with a full circadian mismatch, especially when it crosses multiple time zones or involves a departure in the evening and an arrival in the morning. The result is often a familiar kind of confusion: you may be physically tired, but your brain is still following the old schedule. That is why travel sleep problems are not just about discomfort on the plane or a bad night in a hotel. They are about the body trying to interpret a new day while still living by the timing of the old one.

The direction of travel matters. Flying east usually asks the body to sleep earlier than it wants to, which can feel like a shortened day and an unexpectedly early bedtime. Flying west usually asks the body to stay awake later, which is often easier for many people in the short term but can still produce early morning waking or a stretched-out feeling the next day. When travel crosses only one or two time zones, the body may adapt within a few days if the timing cues are consistent. With larger shifts, the mismatch can last longer, and the first few nights often decide whether the adjustment goes smoothly or gets dragged out by irregular light exposure and inconsistent sleep timing.

One of the most useful ways to reduce the strain is to begin adjusting before departure when possible. If you are traveling east, moving bedtime and wake time a little earlier for several days can make the destination feel less abrupt. If you are traveling west, shifting later can help the body tolerate the longer evening. Even a modest change can help if it is paired with the right light exposure and a stable wake time. The goal is not to fully live in the destination time zone before you leave. It is to narrow the gap so the body does not have to make such a large leap all at once.

Light is especially important during travel because it can either speed adaptation or slow it down. Morning light in the destination time zone helps anchor the new day, while bright light at the wrong time can push the clock in the opposite direction. That means the first morning after arrival is often more important than people realize. Getting outside soon after waking can help the body register the new local time more quickly. At the same time, late-night brightness from airport terminals, hotel lighting, and screens can keep the clock from advancing or delaying in the direction you need. If you arrive in the evening, dimming light and reducing stimulation can make it easier to sleep at the local bedtime rather than stretching the old schedule further.

Sleep on the plane can help, but it helps most when it is used strategically. A long nap at the wrong time can reduce sleep pressure and make the first night in the new location harder. If you need to sleep during travel, aim for a period that supports the destination schedule rather than the departure schedule. For example, if you are trying to adjust to a later time zone, some in-flight sleep may be useful. If you are trying to adjust to an earlier one, sleeping too much during the flight can leave you less ready for the earlier bedtime you need after arrival. The same principle applies to caffeine. It can be useful for staying alert during the hours when you need wakefulness, but too much or too late can make the body hold onto the old rhythm longer than necessary.

Meals and movement can also act as stabilizers. Eating at roughly the local mealtimes helps the body begin treating the destination as the new reference point. A breakfast that is delayed by several hours, or a late-night heavy meal that follows the old time zone, can confuse the timing system and make adaptation less efficient. Light activity after arrival can help with alertness in the daytime and reduce the temptation to collapse too early. Then, once evening comes, the body needs a clear signal that the active part of the day is ending. That means avoiding the common travel pattern of an exhausted daytime nap followed by a late-night stretch of screens, snacks, and irregular wakefulness.

It also helps to decide in advance which adjustment you are making and which one you are not. Many travelers accidentally try to follow both time zones at once: they eat on the new schedule, stay up on the old one, nap whenever fatigue hits, and then wonder why sleep feels scattered. A better approach is to choose the destination clock as soon as you can and support it with repeated cues. That may mean going to bed earlier than feels natural, or staying awake when you would normally doze off, but the point is to send the body one clear message instead of several conflicting ones. After a day or two, the mismatch usually begins to soften if the cues stay consistent.

For frequent travelers, the most effective plan is often not perfection but predictability. Keep wake time as steady as the trip allows, seek bright light at the local morning, reduce light at the local evening, eat meals on the destination schedule, and avoid using naps as a substitute for a full night of sleep unless they are clearly helping you bridge the transition. When travel is brief, you may not fully reset at all, and that is acceptable. The aim is to limit how far the clock drifts and to make the return to normal easier. When travel is longer, the same habits help the body settle more quickly into the new time zone instead of spending several days caught between two different clocks.

Working around shift work and unavoidable night hours

Shift work is difficult for circadian rhythm because it asks the body to do two things that do not fit together: stay alert when the brain expects night, and sleep when the brain expects day. The problem is not only the hours themselves. It is the way those hours collide with light, meals, family obligations, noise, and the natural rise and fall of sleep pressure. If you work nights or rotating shifts, the goal is usually not to make your body clock behave exactly like a daytime schedule. In many cases, that is unrealistic. The more practical aim is to reduce the amount of conflict between your work demands and your body's timing signals so that you can protect sleep, limit exhaustion, and keep the schedule from becoming more disruptive than it has to be.

One of the first decisions to make is whether you are trying to adapt partially to nights or simply survive them with as little circadian damage as possible. Those are not the same strategy. Some people do better by keeping a mostly nocturnal pattern during a stretch of night shifts, especially if the schedule is stable for several days in a row. Others do better by preserving a daytime anchor sleep and using naps, strategic light exposure, and careful timing to get through the work period. The best approach depends on how many nights you work, whether those nights are consecutive, how quickly the schedule changes, and how much control you have over your environment. What matters most is consistency. A repeating night pattern is easier for the body to learn than a schedule that flips back and forth every few days.

If you are on a stable block of night shifts, it can help to treat your sleep period as a protected appointment rather than a flexible leftover. That means deciding in advance when you will sleep after work, how long you will sleep, and what you will do to reduce interruptions. Many night workers do better with a short post-shift sleep followed by a longer sleep period later, while others need one consolidated daytime sleep block. There is no universal formula, but there is a universal principle: the body sleeps better when the timing is repeatable. Even small improvements matter, such as darkening the room, limiting household interruptions, and keeping the phone silent during your protected sleep window. These steps do not erase the circadian mismatch, but they reduce the number of obstacles that keep daytime sleep shallow and fragmented.

Light is one of the most important tools for night work, but it has to be used with intention. Bright light during the night shift can help you stay alert while you are working, especially in the first half of the shift. At the same time, light after the shift can make it harder to fall asleep during the day. That means the timing of light exposure matters as much as the amount. If possible, use bright light while you are on duty and then reduce light on the way home. Sunglasses can help limit morning light exposure after an overnight shift, and keeping your bedroom as dark as possible can make daytime sleep more achievable. For some workers, even a short exposure to morning sunlight on the commute home is enough to delay sleep or make it lighter. That is why the hours immediately after work are often the most important ones to manage carefully.

Meal timing also deserves attention. Night shifts often lead to scattered eating: a large dinner before work, vending machine snacks during the shift, a heavy meal after work, and irregular food intake on days off. That pattern can confuse the body's timing system and make fatigue feel worse. A more stable plan is usually easier on the circadian system. Some workers do well with a main meal before the shift, a lighter meal or snack during the shift, and a small, nonstimulating snack after work if needed before sleep. The goal is not perfection or strict dieting. It is to avoid giving the body constant mixed signals about whether it is daytime or nighttime biology. When meals happen at wildly different hours from one shift to the next, the body has less chance to settle into a usable rhythm.

Rotating schedules are harder than fixed night work because the body never gets enough repetition to adapt fully. If your shifts change from days to evenings to nights, or if your nights are broken up by days off that pull you back toward daytime living, the best strategy is often damage control rather than full adjustment. In that situation, trying to reset completely after every change may create more strain than benefit. Instead, it can help to preserve a few stable anchors that remain as constant as possible: a protected sleep opportunity, a consistent pre-sleep routine, and a predictable pattern for light and meals. Even if the shift itself changes, those anchors give the body something to recognize. For many people, the less they swing between extremes on days off, the easier it is to tolerate the rotating schedule without feeling constantly jet-lagged.

It is also important to plan for the social and practical pressures that make night work harder than it looks on paper. Family needs, errands, appointments, and social expectations can all pull you back into daytime availability just when your body is trying to recover. If you do not protect your sleep, the schedule will usually protect itself by making you more tired, more irritable, and less alert at work. That is why boundaries matter. You may need to decline morning commitments after a shift, keep your sleep room off-limits during certain hours, or use a repeatable routine that tells others when you are unavailable. Night work is not only a test of stamina; it is a test of whether your environment can support the timing demands you are being asked to live under.

There are limits, of course. Some people can adapt reasonably well to certain night schedules, while others remain chronically misaligned no matter how carefully they manage light, sleep, and meals. If you are consistently struggling with insomnia during the day, severe sleepiness on duty, or a pattern that becomes worse with each rotation, that is a sign to re-evaluate rather than simply push harder. The aim is not to prove that you can tolerate an unnatural schedule indefinitely. The aim is to create the safest, most workable version of it, while recognizing that some schedules are inherently hostile to circadian health and may require medical guidance, workplace adjustments, or a different long-term plan.

Recovering after setbacks without starting over

A setback does not erase circadian progress unless you let it become a complete schedule collapse. One late night, one travel day, one emergency, or one stretch of poor sleep can make it feel as if the body clock has snapped back to its old pattern. In reality, the system usually has more memory than that. Circadian timing is built from repeated signals, so a brief disruption may blur the rhythm without fully resetting it. The key is to respond to the interruption in a way that protects the cues you have already established instead of abandoning them out of frustration.

The first temptation after a bad night is to compensate aggressively. People often sleep in for hours, nap longer than usual, go to bed much earlier than planned, or use extra caffeine to power through the day. Those reactions make sense emotionally, but they can create a second problem on top of the first. Sleeping late can weaken the wake-time anchor. Long naps can reduce sleep pressure before night arrives. Going to bed too early can lead to lying awake and associating bedtime with effort instead of sleep. Heavy caffeine use can push the next night later or make sleep lighter. The result is not just recovery from one bad night; it is a new wave of mixed signals.

A better approach is to think in terms of damage control. Preserve the strongest anchors you can, even if the rest of the day is imperfect. If your wake time is already set, keep it as close as possible to normal. If morning light is part of your routine, still get it. If meals are usually timed consistently, keep the first meal and dinner near their usual hours. If you use a wind-down routine, return to it that night even if the day felt chaotic. These small acts may seem too ordinary to matter, but they help the brain recognize that the disruption is temporary and that the underlying pattern still stands.

When sleep is shortened or broken, the goal is not to "make up" the entire loss in one day. The body usually responds better to a steadier correction. If you need to nap, keep it brief and earlier in the day when possible. A short nap can reduce dangerous sleepiness and improve functioning without stealing too much pressure from the next night. If you are dealing with a late schedule after a special event or travel, resist the urge to keep pushing bedtime later for several nights in a row just because the first night was bad. One off-night is a disruption; several unstructured nights can become a new pattern.

It also helps to separate a temporary setback from a true return of the underlying disorder. A person recovering from jet lag may feel off for a few days and then gradually realign as light, meals, and sleep timing settle back into place. Someone with delayed sleep phase may notice that a single late night makes the clock drift later again, but the same correction tools that worked before can still work now. The difference is usually not whether the setback happened, but how quickly you re-establish the signals that move the clock in the right direction. If you respond early, the recovery is often much easier than it feels in the moment.

Another useful habit is to avoid moralizing the setback. A disrupted night is not proof that you failed, and it is not a reason to abandon the entire plan. Circadian work is more like steering than switching. A small turn in the wrong direction can be corrected if you notice it soon enough. If you wake up later than intended, do not treat the whole day as ruined. Use the remaining hours to reinforce the next best timing cue. If you go to bed later than planned, return to the regular wake time rather than extending sleep far into the morning. The system usually recovers faster from one imperfect day than from a series of overreactions.

For people with unstable schedules, it can help to have a "reset floor" rather than a perfect ideal. This is the minimum set of behaviors that keeps the clock from sliding too far: a consistent wake time within a reasonable range, some morning light, meals that are not wildly delayed, and a predictable bedtime routine. On hard days, you may not manage every part of the plan, but meeting the floor is still progress. That approach prevents the all-or-nothing mindset that turns one missed target into a whole lost week.

Most importantly, recovery works best when it is immediate and calm. The sooner you return to the usual anchors, the less opportunity the disruption has to spread. That does not require perfection, only consistency. A setback is information, not a reset button. It tells you where your routine is vulnerable and which cues matter most when life gets messy. If you protect those cues instead of starting over, you give the circadian system the chance to re-stabilize without having to relearn the whole pattern from scratch.

Chapter 9: Working With Clinicians and Treatments

Even with careful light management, consistent routines, and well-chosen habits, some sleep problems need a clinician's perspective to sort out what is driving the pattern and what kind of help is most likely to work. This is especially true when sleep timing is only one part of a broader picture that may include persistent fatigue, snoring, mood changes, medication effects, or a pattern that has resisted self-directed efforts for a long time. Working with a sleep specialist or other clinician does not mean your own observations are unimportant; it means those observations can be used more effectively when they are matched with the right evaluation and treatment approach.

When to seek medical evaluation

Most circadian rhythm sleep problems can be addressed with careful scheduling, light management, and behavior changes, but there are times when self-guided efforts are not enough. Medical evaluation is worth seeking when the pattern is persistent, severe, confusing, or accompanied by other symptoms that suggest something beyond a timing problem alone. The goal is not to turn every sleep struggle into a medical emergency. It is to recognize when the pattern has moved past ordinary circadian misalignment and needs a broader look.

A useful rule is to seek evaluation when sleep timing problems are interfering with daily life in a sustained way. If you are repeatedly unable to fall asleep until very late, waking far too early, or missing work, school, family responsibilities, or social obligations because of sleep timing, that level of disruption deserves attention. The same is true if you have tried consistent wake times, light timing, and routine changes for several weeks without meaningful improvement. Circadian disorders often respond slowly, but they should usually show some direction of change when the timing signals are well matched. If nothing is shifting, the diagnosis may need to be reconsidered, or another condition may be part of the picture.

It is especially important to be evaluated if your sleep pattern is not simply delayed or advanced, but fragmented, unpredictable, or unstable in a way that does not fit a clear circadian pattern. For example, falling asleep and waking at very different times from day to day, sleeping in short pieces across the 24-hour period, or being unable to maintain any regular rhythm may point to a different sleep disorder, a medical issue, medication effects, or a psychiatric condition that is affecting sleep. Circadian rhythm disorders are about timing. When the pattern becomes chaotic rather than consistently shifted, a clinician should help sort out what is driving it.

Other symptoms are also a reason to get checked. Loud snoring, gasping, witnessed pauses in breathing, morning headaches, dry mouth, or excessive daytime sleepiness can suggest sleep apnea or another breathing-related sleep disorder. Restless legs, uncomfortable leg sensations at night, or an urge to move the legs can point to a movement disorder that disrupts sleep onset. Persistent pain, reflux, frequent urination, hot flashes, tremor, palpitations, or unexplained weight change can all interfere with sleep and may require medical treatment in their own right. If sleep is being repeatedly interrupted by something physical, it is better to identify that cause than to keep adjusting bedtime as if timing alone were the problem.

Mood and cognitive changes deserve attention as well. Depression, anxiety, bipolar disorder, attention problems, and some neurodevelopmental conditions can all alter sleep timing, and sleep disruption can also worsen those conditions. If you notice that your sleep pattern is tied to significant mood swings, racing thoughts, unusual energy, panic, hopelessness, or a marked change in behavior, evaluation should not wait. A circadian problem can coexist with a mental health condition, but the treatment approach may need to address both. The same is true if sleep loss is leading to unsafe driving, errors at work, falling asleep in dangerous situations, or a level of irritability and impairment that feels out of proportion to the amount of sleep you are getting.

Medication and substance effects are another reason to involve a clinician. Many common prescriptions and over-the-counter products can shift sleep timing, fragment sleep, or create daytime sleepiness. Stimulants, antidepressants, steroids, decongestants, thyroid medication, pain medicines, and some supplements can all change how alert or sleepy you feel and when that happens. Alcohol can also make sleep seem easier at first while worsening sleep quality later in the night. If your sleep problem began after starting, stopping, or changing a medication, or if you are using melatonin and are unsure whether the timing is helping or hurting, a medical review can prevent you from chasing the wrong solution.

There are also situations where the pattern itself suggests a need for expert guidance. If you suspect a delayed or advanced sleep phase disorder but your schedule is so extreme that ordinary adjustments are not working, a sleep specialist can help confirm the pattern and refine treatment. If you are a shift worker who cannot avoid night hours, a clinician can help you reduce the health cost of an unavoidable schedule. If you travel frequently across time zones and recovery takes much longer than expected, or if you have had a long-standing sleep pattern that has resisted every reasonable attempt to reset it, formal evaluation can clarify whether you are dealing with a circadian disorder, another sleep disorder, or both.

Seek prompt medical attention sooner rather than later if sleep problems are accompanied by chest pain, shortness of breath, fainting, severe confusion, hallucinations, suicidal thoughts, or a sudden and dramatic change in functioning. Those are not routine sleep complaints. They may signal an urgent medical or psychiatric issue that needs immediate care. Even when the situation is less acute, a clinician can help you move from guesswork to a more precise plan. The most useful time to ask for help is not after months of frustration have hardened into discouragement, but when the pattern has become clear enough to see that it is not resolving on its own.

How melatonin timing differs from melatonin dose

Melatonin is often discussed as if it were a sleep pill, but that is only part of the story. In circadian treatment, melatonin is used less for its sedating effect and more for its ability to signal time to the brain. That distinction matters because the amount you take and the time you take it do not do the same job. A higher dose does not necessarily move the body clock more effectively, and a lower dose can still be useful if it is taken at the right point in the daily cycle. For many people, the timing is the treatment; the dose is only the delivery method.

The body responds to melatonin as a message about night. When melatonin rises naturally in the evening, it helps support the transition from daytime alertness to nighttime biology. Supplemental melatonin can reinforce or shift that message, but the effect depends on where your clock is when the signal arrives. Taken at the right time, melatonin can help move the circadian system earlier or support sleep onset. Taken at the wrong time, it may do little, or it may push timing in the wrong direction. That is why two people can take the same dose and have very different results, and why the same person can respond differently depending on whether the goal is to advance, delay, or simply stabilize sleep timing.

Dose refers to how much melatonin is in the tablet, capsule, gummy, or liquid you take. Timing refers to when you take it relative to your internal clock and your target sleep schedule. These are related, but they are not interchangeable. A larger dose may make you feel more drowsy, but drowsiness is not the same as circadian shifting. In fact, a strong sleepy feeling can sometimes mask the real issue by making it seem as if the melatonin is "working" when the clock itself has not moved much. If the goal is to change the timing of sleep, you want to think first about the signal being sent to the brain, not just the intensity of the sensation.

This is one reason low doses are often favored in circadian use. Many people assume that more is better, especially when sleep has been difficult for a long time. But melatonin does not behave like a typical medication where a stronger dose necessarily produces a stronger benefit. For timing purposes, very small amounts may be enough to communicate the evening signal the brain needs. Higher doses can linger longer, increase next-morning grogginess, or create a heavier sedative effect that is not especially helpful if you are trying to shift your clock rather than simply knock yourself out. The aim is usually to provide a clear cue, not to overwhelm the system.

Timing also determines whether melatonin is being used as a sleep aid, a circadian shifter, or both. If you take it close to bedtime, you may be using it mainly to support sleep onset. If you take it earlier in the evening, you may be using it to nudge the body clock toward an earlier schedule. That earlier timing is often the more important strategy for delayed sleep patterns, because the brain needs repeated advance signals before it begins to expect sleep sooner. For advanced sleep patterns, melatonin timing may need to be handled very differently, and in some cases it may not be appropriate at all without clinician guidance. The key point is that the same substance can serve different purposes depending on when it is taken.

People sometimes make the mistake of adjusting the dose when what they really need to adjust is the clock-time of administration. If a small dose seems ineffective, the answer is not always to increase it. It may be that the timing is too late to produce a meaningful circadian effect, or too early to match the intended goal. Likewise, if melatonin makes you feel too sleepy or foggy, the solution may be to lower the dose rather than abandon the treatment entirely. The right balance is often found by separating two questions: How much melatonin is enough to create the signal? And when should that signal be delivered for the type of shift you need?

Because melatonin is a timing cue, consistency matters here as well. Taking it at roughly the same time each evening helps the body recognize the pattern, just as consistent light exposure and wake time do. Irregular use can weaken the message and make it harder to tell whether the treatment is helping. It also helps to remember that melatonin works best as part of a broader plan. A carefully chosen dose taken at the wrong time, while bright evening light is still pouring in and wake time is drifting later on weekends, is unlikely to produce much change. The clock responds to the combined pattern, not to one isolated action.

For that reason, melatonin is usually most useful when it is treated as one timed signal among several. The goal is not to chase sleep with a stronger and stronger dose, but to use the smallest effective amount at the right point in the day, while keeping the rest of the schedule aligned with the shift you want. When the timing is right, melatonin can help the body recognize night more clearly. When the dose is right as well, the signal is often cleaner, more tolerable, and more likely to support the larger circadian plan.

Behavioral treatment options and sleep coaching

Behavioral treatment is often the foundation of circadian care because it changes the conditions that keep the clock drifting in the first place. Light therapy can push timing in one direction, but daily behavior determines whether that shift holds. In practice, behavioral treatment is less about trying harder and more about reducing the mixed signals that make the brain uncertain about when day ends and night begins. That can include stabilizing wake time, limiting time in bed to what the body can actually use for sleep, building a predictable wind-down, and changing the habits that quietly reinforce the wrong schedule. When these elements are coordinated, sleep often becomes less of a nightly negotiation and more of a learned pattern the body can follow.

One of the most useful behavioral approaches is called sleep scheduling or sleep restriction, though the name can sound harsher than the method really is. The idea is not to deprive you of sleep. It is to narrow the amount of time spent in bed so that sleep has a stronger chance of consolidating. Many people with circadian rhythm problems spend extra hours in bed trying to force sleep, only to teach the body that bed is a place for wakefulness, frustration, and clock-watching. A sleep coach or clinician may help determine a realistic sleep window based on your actual sleep pattern, then adjust it gradually as sleep becomes more efficient. This approach can be especially helpful when delayed timing has been paired with long periods of lying awake.

Stimulus control is another core behavior change. It teaches the brain to reconnect the bed with sleep rather than with alertness. That usually means using the bed only for sleep and intimacy, getting out of bed if you are awake and restless for too long, and returning only when sleepiness is clearly present. For someone who has spent months or years trying to “make” sleep happen, this can feel counterintuitive at first. Yet the logic is straightforward: if the bed becomes the place where you practice being awake, the brain learns wakefulness there. If it becomes the place where sleep reliably occurs, the brain begins to treat it as a cue for shutdown. A coach can help you apply this without becoming rigid or discouraged by occasional rough nights.

Sleep coaching adds structure to these behavioral tools. A good coach does more than hand out rules. The coach helps translate general principles into a schedule that fits your life, monitors what is and is not changing, and adjusts the plan when real-world demands interfere. That matters because circadian treatment often fails when people receive advice that is technically correct but impossible to sustain. Someone working early shifts, caring for children, or recovering from chronic sleep debt may need a different sequence of changes than someone with a stable schedule and a delayed sleep phase pattern. Coaching can also help identify the hidden behaviors that keep the clock unstable, such as irregular weekend sleep, late-night food, excessive time in bed, or inconsistent morning routines.

Cognitive behavioral therapy for insomnia, often called CBT-I, is frequently adapted for circadian rhythm problems when insomnia has become part of the picture. Many people with a body clock disorder also develop conditioned insomnia: they begin to associate nighttime with effort, fear, and disappointment. CBT-I addresses that learned pattern by changing sleep-related thoughts and behaviors, reducing the tendency to lie awake in bed, and rebuilding confidence in the body’s ability to sleep. For someone with circadian misalignment, CBT-I is most helpful when it is used alongside timing-based treatment rather than as a substitute for it.

If the clock is still pulling sleep in the wrong direction, behavioral work alone may not be enough. But when the timing cues are being corrected, CBT-I can remove the extra layer of anxiety and hyperarousal that keeps sleep from settling.

Relaxation strategies also belong in behavioral treatment, but they work best as support rather than as the main event. Breathing exercises, progressive muscle relaxation, guided imagery, and mindfulness practices can lower the arousal that keeps sleep at arm's length. They are useful because a person with a circadian disorder often becomes conditioned to expect struggle at bedtime. The goal is not to "force relaxation," which can become its own kind of pressure, but to create a predictable transition from active evening to sleep-ready night. A calm routine repeated in the same order can become a cue in itself. Over time, the body begins to associate those steps with the end of the day, which makes the transition less abrupt.

Sleep coaching is also valuable because it helps with adherence, and adherence is where many circadian plans break down. It is one thing to understand that wake time should stay fixed, that naps should be limited, or that you should leave bed when sleep will not come. It is another thing to do those things consistently when you are tired, stressed, or discouraged. A coach can help you problem-solve around the predictable obstacles: social events that run late, mornings that start too early, weekends that tempt you to "catch up," and setbacks that make you want to abandon the plan. The point is not perfection. The point is to keep the overall pattern moving in the right direction often enough for the body to recognize it.

For many people, the best results come when behavioral treatment is treated as a system rather than a list of tips. Fixed wake time, limited time in bed, stimulus control, consistent evening routines, and support for anxiety or frustration all work on the same problem from different angles. A sleep coach helps you decide which piece matters most first, because the order can matter. Someone with severe delayed sleep may need timing and light changes before strict sleep restriction makes sense. Someone with advanced sleep phase may need a different set of anchors to keep evenings from collapsing too early. The value of behavioral treatment is that it can be tailored, measured, and refined. It gives you a way to work with the clock instead of fighting it one night at a time.

Questions to ask a sleep specialist

When you meet with a sleep specialist, the most useful questions are the ones that turn a vague complaint into a clear clinical picture. You are not just trying to prove that your sleep is difficult; you are trying to help the clinician identify whether the problem is truly circadian, whether another sleep disorder is involved, and which treatment approach fits your pattern. A good visit is less about describing how tired you are and more about showing how your sleep behaves across time. That usually means asking about the pattern itself, the timing of symptoms, and the logic behind each recommendation.

Start by asking what diagnosis best fits your pattern and what else needs to be ruled out. If you are told you may have delayed sleep phase, advanced sleep phase, shift work disorder, or another circadian problem, ask what features support that conclusion. Ask what findings would make the specialist consider insomnia, sleep apnea, restless legs, depression, medication effects, or another condition instead. This matters because circadian disorders can coexist with other problems, and treating the wrong layer first can leave you frustrated. A useful question is: "What makes you think this is a circadian timing issue rather than only a sleep-onset or sleep-maintenance problem?"

It is also worth asking how the diagnosis was made and whether more information is needed. Some specialists rely heavily on your history and a sleep diary; others may recommend actigraphy, a sleep study, or additional testing depending on the case. Ask, “What data would help you confirm the pattern?” and “Do you need me to track sleep, light exposure, naps, meals, or work hours before the next visit?” If you have already been tracking your sleep, bring that record and ask how the clinician interprets it. The goal is to make sure the treatment plan is based on your actual timing pattern, not on a single rough estimate of your bedtime.

Once the pattern is clear, ask about the treatment plan in terms of timing, not just medication names. For example, if melatonin is suggested, ask why it is being used, what time it should be taken, and what result it is supposed to produce. Ask whether the goal is to shift the clock earlier, make sleep easier, or both. If light therapy is part of the plan, ask when to use it, how bright it should be, how long each session should last, and what to do on days when your schedule changes. A helpful question is: “What is the timing target for this treatment, and how will we know if it is moving my clock in the right direction?”

You should also ask what the plan expects you to do every day, because circadian treatment depends on consistency. Ask which habits matter most: wake time, bedtime, morning light, evening light reduction, meal timing, exercise timing, or something else. If the specialist gives several recommendations, ask which one has the highest priority if you cannot do everything at once. That question can prevent the common mistake of trying to change too many variables at the same time. You might ask, “If I can only focus on one or two anchors first, which ones will make the biggest difference?”

Another important topic is safety and side effects. Ask whether any treatment could make you too sleepy, too alert, or otherwise worse before it gets better. If melatonin is part of the plan, ask about possible morning grogginess, vivid dreams, interactions with other medications, and whether the dose matters as much as the timing. If light therapy is recommended, ask whether there are any reasons you should avoid it, especially if you have eye disease, bipolar disorder, migraines, or a history of mood changes related to light exposure. A good specialist should be willing to explain both the benefits and the limits of the approach. You are looking for a plan that is effective and realistic, not one that sounds simple but ignores your medical context.

It also helps to ask how progress will be measured. Circadian treatment can be subtle, and people often expect an immediate transformation when the real change happens in stages. Ask what improvements should come first: falling asleep earlier, waking with less effort, fewer nighttime awakenings, better daytime alertness, or more stable energy across the week. Ask how long the specialist expects it to take before the treatment shows a meaningful effect, and when you should report back if nothing is changing. A useful question is: "What would count as progress in the first two weeks, and what would tell us this plan needs to be adjusted?"

If your schedule is unusual, ask how the plan should adapt to real life. Shift work, travel, parenting, school, and rotating obligations can all interfere with a standard circadian plan. Ask what to do on days off, after a night shift, after crossing time zones, or when you have to wake earlier than usual. Ask whether the specialist recommends a stable long-term schedule or a flexible strategy built around your work demands. The more specific the question, the more useful the answer will be: "How should I apply this plan on workdays versus days off?" or "What should I do differently when my schedule changes for only a few days?"

Finally, ask what the next step is if the first plan does not work. That question is not pessimistic; it is practical. Circadian disorders often require adjustment, and a good clinician should expect that. Ask whether the plan would be changed by altering light timing, melatonin timing, sleep schedule anchors, or another part of the routine. Ask how many attempts are reasonable before reconsidering the diagnosis. The point is to leave the appointment knowing not only what to do, but also what to watch for and how the treatment will evolve if your body does not respond the way the first plan predicts.

Conclusion

The work of resetting a circadian rhythm is rarely dramatic in the moment. More often, it is a series of small corrections that begin to add up: a steadier wake time, a brighter morning, a quieter evening, a more predictable first meal, a bedtime that stops drifting farther and farther away. None of those changes feels as powerful as a single perfect night of sleep, but the body does not reset on promises or intentions. It resets on repeated signals that arrive at the right time.

That is why progress can be easy to miss while it is happening. You may not notice the clock moving by minutes at first. You may only notice that getting out of bed is less punishing, that sleepiness arrives with a little more order, or that the late-night second wind no longer takes over quite as often. These are not minor details. They are signs that the system is beginning to trust the pattern you are building.

There will also be days when the pattern seems to disappear. Travel, illness, stress, family demands, late work, and ordinary life can all interrupt the rhythm you have been trying to establish. That does not mean the effort failed. Circadian timing is not fragile in the sense that one disruption destroys everything, but it is sensitive enough that repeated inconsistency can blur the message. When that happens, the answer is usually not to start over from zero. It is to return to the most reliable anchors and let them do their work again.

For many people, the hardest part is not learning what to do. It is believing that small, ordinary actions can be strong enough to change sleep. Yet the body clock is built from exactly those kinds of actions. Light at the right time, a wake time that does not move, meals that happen in a regular window, and a wind-down that repeats in the same order each night all tell the brain the same thing: this is the shape of the day. Over time, that message becomes biology.

Some readers will discover that their sleep problem is mostly a matter of timing and can be improved with consistency and patience. Others will find that behavior changes help, but not enough on their own, because another sleep disorder, medication effect, medical issue, or work constraint is also part of the picture. Both experiences are valid. The goal is not to force every sleep problem into the same solution. The goal is to understand what is driving your pattern and respond to it with the right tools.

If you have spent a long time feeling as though your sleep is controlled by chance, the most important shift may be this: circadian rhythm is not fixed fate, and it is not a moral test. It is a timing system that can be influenced. That influence is strongest when the signals you send are simple, repeatable, and aligned with the direction you want the clock to move. The more consistent those signals become, the less sleep has to rely on guesswork.

Resetting your clock is not about becoming perfect with sleep. It is about making the next day easier for your body to recognize than the one before. When that happens, sleep stops feeling like something you must chase and starts becoming something your system knows how to approach.

Appendix: Practical Tools and Tracking Templates

At this point, the most useful thing you can do is make the process visible. Sleep problems that feel chaotic on the inside often become easier to work with once they are written down, compared, and reviewed in a consistent way. The tools in this appendix are meant to support that kind of clarity without turning your day into a data-collection project. They give you a structured place to notice patterns, track timing cues, and keep your plan simple enough to follow in real life. If you have been trying to remember what happened last night, or whether this week is actually better than the one before it, these pages can help you answer those questions with less guesswork. Use them as working documents, not tests. The point is to gather enough information to guide your next adjustment and to make your circadian pattern easier to see when you look back over time.

Sleep and energy diary template

A sleep and energy diary works best when it is simple enough that you will actually use it every day. The purpose is not to create a perfect research record. It is to capture the timing pattern of your sleep, alertness, and daily cues in a way that makes drift, consistency, and triggers easier to see. If you have been trying to understand why some days feel reasonably stable while others feel out of control, a diary can turn vague impressions into something you can compare across time.

Keep the format brief. For most people, one page per day is enough. Use the same categories each day so the record stays easy to scan later. At minimum, note when you went to bed, when you think you fell asleep, how many times you woke during the night, when you finally got out of bed, and how rested or alert you felt on waking. Add a simple daytime energy rating at a few points in the day, such as morning, afternoon, and evening. A 1-to-5 scale is usually enough, where 1 means very low energy and 5 means very high energy. The goal is not precision down to the minute; it is pattern recognition.

Include the timing cues that may be influencing your clock. Write down when you first saw bright outdoor light, whether you used a light box, when you dimmed lights in the evening, and how much screen time you had close to bedtime. Also note meal times, caffeine, alcohol, exercise, naps, and anything unusual such as travel, illness, stress, or a late social event. These details matter because sleep timing is rarely shaped by one factor alone. Often it is the combination of a late meal, bright evening light, and a nap after dinner that pushes sleep later, or an early wake time, morning light, and regular meals that support a more stable rhythm.

Use plain language. You do not need to describe every hour of the day. A few honest notes are more useful than a long record you abandon after three days. For example: "Woke at 6:45 a.m. with alarm, energy 2/5, sleepy after lunch, nap 20 minutes at 3:00 p.m., caffeine at 9:00 a.m. and 1:30 p.m., screens until 11:15 p.m., lights out 11:30 p.m., slept around midnight." That kind of entry gives you enough information to see whether your sleep is drifting later, whether daytime sleepiness is building at the same time each day, and whether certain habits are reinforcing the pattern.

If you want the diary to be especially useful for circadian work, track the same items in the same order every day. Consistency makes comparison easier. A simple structure can look like this:

Bedtime: when you got into bed

Sleep onset: estimated time you fell asleep

Night awakenings: number and approximate duration

Wake time: when you got out of bed for the day

Energy ratings: morning, afternoon, evening

Light exposure: outdoor light, light box, bright indoor light, screens

Meals and caffeine: timing of first meal, lunch, dinner, caffeine cutoff

Movement: exercise, walk outside, unusually sedentary day

Disruptions: nap, travel, stress, pain, alcohol, shift change

Do not worry if your estimates are imperfect. Many people do not know exactly when they fell asleep, and that is normal. If you are unsure, write "estimated" rather than trying to force certainty. Over time, the value of the diary comes less from any single day and more from repeated patterns. You may notice that your best energy days follow a morning light routine, or that sleep becomes lighter after late caffeine, or that your weekend wake time shifts enough to make Monday feel like jet lag. Those observations are often more useful than an exact sleep latency number.

It can also help to add one short sentence at the end of each day about how the day felt overall. For example: "Felt foggy until noon, then better after a walk outside," or "Alert late at night despite feeling tired earlier." This kind of note captures the mismatch between sleep drive and circadian timing that numbers alone can miss. If you are working with a clinician, these brief comments can be especially helpful because they show how the pattern affects function, not just how many hours you spent in bed.

Finally, keep the diary where it fits naturally into your routine. Some people prefer paper on the nightstand. Others do better with a phone note or a simple spreadsheet. The best format is the one you can maintain without turning it into another source of stress. If you miss a day, resume the next day without trying to reconstruct everything perfectly. A useful diary is not the one with the most detail. It is the one that stays honest, repeatable, and clear enough to show how your body clock is behaving across ordinary days.

Light exposure and screen-time checklist

Use this checklist to make your light habits more deliberate and less accidental. The goal is not to live in darkness or to chase brightness all day long. It is to notice when light is helping your clock and when it is quietly working against the timing you are trying to build. Because light is such a strong circadian signal, small changes in when and how you encounter it can matter more than people expect.

Morning light: Within the first hour after waking, aim to get bright outdoor light if possible. A short walk, standing outside with coffee, or even sitting near a sunny window can help, but outdoor light is usually much stronger than indoor light. If you are trying to shift your schedule earlier, this is one of the most important habits to protect. If mornings are dark where you live or your schedule makes outdoor light difficult, use a light therapy box only as directed and at the correct time for your sleep pattern.

Midday light: Notice whether you are spending most of the day indoors under dim or uneven lighting. A very dim daytime environment can weaken the contrast between day and night, especially if you are already struggling with a delayed rhythm. If possible, add some daylight exposure before late afternoon. This does not need to be a formal therapy session; even ordinary daytime light helps reinforce that the active part of the day is still underway.

Evening light: In the two to three hours before bed, reduce bright light as much as practical. Overhead lighting, bright kitchen lights, and especially screens can keep the brain in a more alert state than you want at night. If your sleep is delayed, evening light reduction is especially important because late light can push your clock later. If your sleep comes too early, the timing may need to be adjusted differently, but the general principle still holds: avoid unnecessary brightness when your body should be transitioning toward sleep.

Screen use: Check whether your screen habits match your sleep goal. Ask yourself:

Do I use phones, tablets, laptops, or TV in bed?

Do I keep scrolling after I notice I am getting sleepy?

Do I use screens in the last hour before sleep without lowering brightness?

Do I feel more alert after reading messages, watching videos, or checking news at night?

If the answer to any of these is yes, the screen itself may be part of the problem, but the content matters too. Emotional or stimulating material can keep you mentally activated even if the light level is modest. For that reason, screen management is not only about blue light filters. It is also about what your attention is doing at the end of the day. If you need a screen at night, lower the brightness, use night mode if it helps, and keep the session as short and calm as possible.

Device settings and environment: Make your light environment easier to control by changing the defaults. Dim the lights in the last part of the evening, keep lamps lower and warmer when you can, and avoid bright overhead lighting after dinner. Put chargers outside the bedroom if possible so the bed does not become a place for extended screen time. If you use a computer late at night, consider whether you can finish the most stimulating work earlier and save only low-demand tasks for later.

Consistency check: Review whether your light pattern changes sharply from weekday to weekend. A strong morning-light habit during the workweek can be weakened if you sleep late and stay indoors on days off. Likewise, a careful evening routine can be undone by a bright, late night out or a long stretch of screen use after midnight. Your clock responds to repeated timing, not to isolated good days, so the most useful checklist item is whether your light exposure is predictable enough to teach the body what time it is.

Daily yes/no review: At the end of the day, it can help to ask yourself a few simple questions and answer honestly:

Did I get outdoor light soon after waking?

Did I spend time in bright light during the day?

Did I lower light levels in the evening?

Did I avoid screens, or at least reduce how late and how intensely I used them?

Did my light habits support the sleep timing I am trying to build?

If you miss a step, do not treat it as failure. Treat it as information. The purpose of the checklist is to show you where the day is helping your circadian rhythm and where it is sending mixed signals. Over time, that awareness makes it easier to adjust the parts of the day that matter most.

Weekly circadian reset planner

A weekly reset planner works best when it turns circadian change into a set of repeatable actions rather than a vague intention to "sleep better." The point is not to create a perfect schedule for seven flawless days. It is to build a week that gives your body the same timing cues often enough for the clock to start trusting them. That means choosing a few anchors that stay steady even when the rest of life is imperfect: wake time, first light, meal timing, evening dimming, and a bedtime window that does not keep drifting. When those anchors repeat, the brain has a better chance of recognizing the pattern and using it to organize sleep.

Start by deciding what you are trying to move. If your sleep is too late, the week should be built around earlier morning cues and a firmer evening cutoff. If your sleep is too early, the week should protect evening light and delay sleepiness without creating a second round of late-night stimulation. If your schedule is unstable because of work, school, or caregiving, the goal may be less about shifting the clock and more about preventing it from swinging wildly. A useful planner always matches the direction of the problem. Otherwise, you can work very hard and still send the wrong signal to the body.

Use the same structure each day so the plan stays readable at a glance. Many people do well with a simple seven-day grid that includes wake time, outdoor light, meals, exercise, caffeine cutoff, screen reduction, and bedtime target. You do not need to fill every box with a perfect performance goal. Instead, mark the one or two behaviors that matter most for your current pattern. For example, someone with delayed sleep phase may focus on getting up at the same time every morning and getting bright light within the first hour of waking. Someone with advanced sleep phase may focus on protecting evening light and avoiding an overly early bedtime. The planner is strongest when it clarifies priorities instead of piling on every possible habit.

It also helps to build the week around your most stable day, not your most difficult one. If weekdays are constrained by work, set the weekday wake time and then keep weekends close to it rather than treating Saturday and Sunday as a separate sleep universe. If your work schedule changes, anchor the plan to the part of the day you can control most reliably, such as the first meal after waking or a fixed light exposure routine. The body clock responds to repetition, so the value of the planner comes from consistency across ordinary days, not from making one day unusually strict and another one unusually loose.

As you use the planner, watch for mixed signals. A common mistake is to make one part of the day more circadian-friendly while another part quietly pulls in the opposite direction. For instance, a person may get morning light but then nap long in the afternoon, drink caffeine late, stay in bright light at night, and wonder why the schedule does not move. Another person may keep evenings dark but sleep in late, missing the morning cue that would help advance the clock. The planner should help you spot those conflicts before they become habits. If the day has too many exceptions, the clock receives too many instructions.

It can be useful to think of the week in terms of "protect," "reduce," and "repeat." Protect the signals that matter most, such as a fixed wake time or a consistent bedtime routine. Reduce the signals that interfere, such as late bright light, irregular naps, or caffeine that lasts into the evening. Repeat the cues that teach the body what time it is, such as the same morning light exposure, the same first meal window, or the same wind-down sequence. That kind of structure keeps the plan practical. You are not trying to micromanage every hour; you are trying to make the important hours predictable enough to reshape timing.

When the week does not go as planned, do not rewrite the whole system from one bad night. A reset planner is meant to absorb ordinary disruptions without collapsing. If you stayed up too late one night, return to the anchor points the next day rather than sleeping in for hours and pushing the whole cycle later. If you had to work late, travel, or deal with an interruption, resume the plan at the next available cue instead of waiting for a "clean start." Circadian change is built from the signals you repeat after the disruption, not from the perfection of the disruption-free week.

Use the planner as a working document, not a test. At the end of the week, compare what you intended with what actually happened and look for patterns that can guide the next seven days. Maybe the wake time held but evening light was harder to control. Maybe meals were steady during the week but drifted on weekends. Maybe one small change, repeated daily, did more than several ambitious changes that never stuck. That information is what makes the planner useful. It helps you see which cues your body is responding to and which ones still need to be simplified, strengthened, or timed more carefully.

Quick-reference guide to common sleep disorder patterns

Sleep disorder patterns are easiest to understand when you look at them as timing signatures rather than isolated complaints. Two people can both say, "I can't sleep," yet one is dealing with a clock that runs late, another with a clock that runs early, and a third with a schedule that changes so often the body never settles long enough to establish a rhythm. The pattern matters because it points toward the kind of intervention that is most likely to help. If you keep treating every sleep problem as the same problem, you can end up using the wrong cue at the wrong time and making the mismatch worse.

A delayed sleep pattern usually looks like a consistent struggle to fall asleep until very late, followed by difficulty waking in the morning. The person is often more alert at night than they want to be and feels most functional later in the day. The key feature is not simply preferring late hours. It is that sleep does not come naturally at a socially useful bedtime, even when the person is trying to sleep. If this pattern is stable across weeks and tends to improve when obligations are removed, it often points toward a delayed circadian phase. In that case, the problem is less about willingness and more about the body clock sending its sleep signal too late.

An advanced sleep pattern is the mirror image in many ways. Sleepiness arrives early in the evening, sometimes so early that the person struggles to stay awake through normal social or family hours. Waking also happens too early, often before the desired rise time, and the person may feel fully alert at a time when they would prefer more sleep. This pattern is easy to miss because it can look like "being a morning person." The difference is that a true advanced pattern is rigid. The person is not simply choosing early nights; the body is repeatedly pushing sleep and wakefulness earlier than the schedule requires.

Shift-work pattern problems usually have a different feel because the issue is not a single internal timing shift so much as repeated conflict between the clock and the schedule. Sleep may be fragmented, shortened, or unrefreshing after night work, and the person may feel sleepy at work, wired after the shift, and then unable to sleep long enough during the day. Rotating schedules can make the pattern even less stable because the body never gets enough repetition to adapt. If the sleep problem improves on days off but returns with each work cycle, that points toward a schedule-driven circadian strain rather than a fixed personal sleep phase.

Jet lag is usually easier to identify because it follows travel. The body feels as if it is living in the old time zone while the environment demands the new one. Sleepiness may arrive at the wrong local hour, waking may happen too early or too late, and appetite, energy, and alertness can feel displaced for several days. The important clue is that the pattern is linked to a recent time-zone change and gradually improves as the body adapts. That makes jet lag different from a chronic circadian disorder, even though the symptoms can feel very similar in the short term.

Irregular sleep-wake patterns are less about being early or late and more about lacking a stable rhythm at all. Bedtime and wake time may vary widely from day to day, sleep may happen in pieces, and there may be no consistent anchor for the body to learn from. This pattern can appear in people with highly unpredictable schedules, but it can also show up when habits, naps, light exposure, and wake times are all changing in ways that prevent the system from settling. The challenge here is not just moving the clock in one direction. It is creating enough regularity for the brain to recognize a day-night structure again.

Not every pattern fits neatly into one box, and that is one reason this guide is meant to be used as a quick reference rather than a diagnosis. The same person can show more than one feature at once. For example, someone may have a delayed pattern during the school year, then develop a more irregular pattern during vacation, then experience jet lag after travel on top of both. What you are looking for is the dominant shape of the problem: late, early, shift-based, travel-based, or scattered. Once the shape is clear, the next question becomes which timing cues are most likely to move it in the right direction.

If you are trying to match your experience to a pattern, these simple distinctions can help:

Delayed pattern: sleep comes much later than desired, waking is difficult, and evenings feel more alert than mornings.

Advanced pattern: sleepiness comes too early, waking comes too early, and late evening hours feel unusually hard to maintain.

Shift-work pattern: sleep and alertness are repeatedly forced out of sync by night work or rotating hours.

Jet lag: symptoms begin after travel across time zones and gradually fade as the body adapts.

Irregular pattern: sleep timing changes so often that the body never settles into a dependable rhythm.

The most useful question is not, "Why can't I sleep?" but, "What timing pattern is this sleep following?" That shift in attention can turn a confusing problem into a recognizable one. Once the pattern is named, the path forward becomes much clearer, because each circadian problem responds best to a different combination of light, schedule, and behavioral cues.

www.ingramcontent.com/pod-product-compliance
Lightning Source LLC
LaVergne TN
LVHW040520210926
848480LV00007BA/1531